The Spirit of MANAAKI

"Born homesick, I am the child of many cultures, displaced and yearning to be rooted in my own ancestral homeland. . . . I felt the hands of Maata were weaving along with my heart and hands a story of redemption, of forgiving, for all the generations of my people who lost their authentic customs and way of life. . . . Thank you, Maata; thank you, Stephanie; thank you, all our ancestors; and all our future generations to come—our love is the revolution of peace on Earth."

IBU ROBIN LIM, FOUNDER OF BUMI SEHAT AND 2011 CNN HERO OF THE YEAR

"*The Spirit of Manaaki* is a rare and welcome creation of integrative storytelling. Stephanie Mines skillfully, humbly, and lovingly bridges our shattered, dominant worldview with the relationally aware and intact Indigenous worldview of the Māori, while centering Maata's guidance for cultivating our own capacities for stewarding life, finding belonging, and forgiving the unforgivable as a path to love of self and others. This journey into the Māori world may sound like 'a step into a distant, or even a fantasy, past, but it is actually a view of the future.'"

LISA REAGAN, FOUNDER OF KINDRED WORLD AND EDITOR OF *KINDRED MAGAZINE*

"*The Spirit of Manaaki* is a profound revelation, an awakening that nurtures hope for real, positive change in your life, the world, and our planet."

ANTONELLA SANSONE, PH.D., CREATOR OF THE PRENATAL MINDFULNESS RELATIONSHIP-BASED PROGRAM

"This book is a reverent offering to Maata Wharehoka and the living legacy of Parihaka—a place where ancestral memory, nonviolent resistance, and cultural sovereignty are tended through daily practice. Through story, ritual, and the weaving of feminine and land-based wisdom, it reveals a vision of leadership rooted not in control, but in sacred reciprocity and collective care."

Allie Davis, Ph.D., maternal ecotherapist and creator of the Mother Tree Method

"If we are to survive these challenging times, we must read *The Spirit of Manaaki* and imbibe the worldview of the elder wisdom of Maata Wharehoka that we desperately need."

Cherionna Menzam-Sills, Ph.D., author of *The Prenatal Shadow*

"Stephanie Mines conveys the story of Maata Wharehoka with reverence and responsibility, offering a bridge between generations, cultures, and worlds in service to a future rooted in ancestral truth. This book is a sacred act of remembrance that transcends the page."

Kristy King, M.D., Regenerative and Environmental Medicine, and women's health advocate

"*The Spirit of Manaaki* contains timeless Māori wisdom that reminds us of universal truths on a profound cellular level. These truths provide the guidance we need to mend what has been broken and move forward together as one human family, creating peace on Earth."

Sierra Sugrue, N.D.

"*The Spirit of Manaaki* is a lyrical catalogue of the impact of a Māori woman rooted in self-determination and dedication to her people. As a Pākehā (settler) woman in Aotearoa (New Zealand) who aspires to become a regenerative health leader, I find the stories and wisdom in this book to be invaluable teachings on my path. I am thrilled to have this book for myself, and appreciate that, through it, Maata's legacy will continue to positively affect the world, reaching ever-widening circles for the benefit of all life."

Chloe Waretini, trauma therapist, Aotearoa

The Spirit of MANAAKI

Maata, a Living Library of Māori Wisdom and Medicine Practices

A Sacred Planet Book

STEPHANIE MINES, Ph.D.

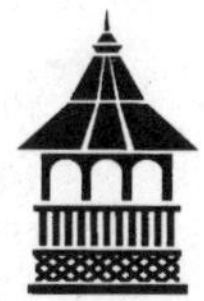

Park Street Press
Rochester, Vermont

Park Street Press
One Park Street
Rochester, Vermont 05767
www.ParkStPress.com

Park Street Press is a division of Inner Traditions International

Sacred Planet Books are curated by Richard Grossinger, Inner Traditions editorial board member and cofounder and former publisher of North Atlantic Books. The Sacred Planet collection, published under the umbrella of the Inner Traditions family of imprints, includes works on the themes of consciousness, cosmology, alternative medicine, dreams, climate, permaculture, alchemy, shamanic studies, oracles, astrology, crystals, hyperobjects, locutions, and subtle bodies.

Cataloging-in-Publication Data for this title is available from the Library of Congress

ISBN 979-8-88850-095-8 (print)
ISBN 979-8-88850-096-5 (ebook)

Printed and bound in the United States by Lake Book Manufacturing, LLC

10 9 8 7 6 5 4 3 2 1

Text design and layout by Priscilla Harris Baker
This book was typeset in Garamond, with Antiquarian Scribe, Gill Sans, and Futura used as display typefaces

To send correspondence to the author of this book, mail a first-class letter to the author c/o Inner Traditions, One Park Street, Rochester, VT 05767, and we will forward the communication, or contact the author directly at **stephaniemines.com**.

This book is dedicated to the children, grandchildren, and great-grandchildren of Maata Wharehoka.

Jean Hikaka, Elias Lilo, Puna Te Aroha Wharehoka, Ngahina Te Reihana Wharehoka, and Atahere Te Akau Wharehoka each carry a portion of Maata's mantle.

Maata's grandchildren and great-grandchildren are Maata's greatest delight. Everything that Maata accomplishes is in their name, for their futures, and for all tangata whenua.

Whitirangihau Hikaka, Rangianewanewa Hikaka, Te Rangihuatau Hikaka, Tukerekere Hikaka, Dallas King, Kingston Lilo, Talei-Jean Lilo, Lennard Lilo, Rongowhakata Greening, Rameka Te Amai Greening, Reign Greening, Rereaio Greening, Te Hoiere Limmer, Mahara i Te Rangi Limmer, Tamarua Te Tuakana Limmer, Herengārangi Wharehoka, Te Ita o Te Rumoana Wharehoka, Kāmairā Wharehoka, Hinemaiora Wano-Ruakere, Hotukura Wharehoka.

Te Raukaerea Hikaka-Koha, Mīere o Te Rangi Hikaka-Karena, Kauri Craig, Kaylen Tui Karena, Leilani Power, Kade Hikaka, Layla-Rose Hikaka, Mya Hikaka, Iluka Hikaka, Micah Hikaka, Izaliyah King, Rehua-Atatu Marriott, Te Kōtuku-Teiria King, Nehemiah-Manuao King.

To all the children who have been loved by Maata, who have sat with Maata, had hugs, and had her kuikui growlings, he mihi tēnei ki a koe.

This book is for you!

Contents

FOREWORD

Manifesting Global Unity

Anita Sanchez, Ph.D.

The mere presence of Māori Elder Maata, whether in person or through her words and spirit, is inspiring. She moves me to love myself, challenge myself, be and do better for myself, for others, and for future generations of our children and the children of other species.

I first heard about Maata Wharehoka in Findhorn, Scotland, at the Climate Change and Consciousness Conference in 2019. Her son, representing Maata and the iconic Parihaka marae where nonviolent activism was born, introduced her to me. Te Akau, along with others from the Taranaki region on the North Island of Aotearoa who came to the conference at Maata's request, embodied the power and dignity that Maata imparted to them. They spoke of her environmental advocacy and, most significantly, of the inspirational guidance they received from their tūpuna (ancestors) at all times. My conversations with them were filled with laughter and candid talks. And while Maata was not physically present, her peaceful, confident knowing of a path forward for her community and for the world has never left me. We are sisters, united as women and as elders, as voices for our living earth, the theme of climate change, and consciousness.

When you read Maata's stories in this book, transcribed via her appointed biographer, Stephanie Mines, Ph.D., you, too, will understand how her powerful model of strong feminine leadership and her undying vision of unity compelled her to continually do her own healing and even forgive the unforgivable. Maata is absolutely clear about this. There are no shortcuts to manifesting this global unity, and there will be no progress forward without it. We share the personal, lived experience of how the essential gift of forgiving the unforgivable must be present to truly attain unity. Maata speaks my language. This is also my message as an Indigenous woman and elder. There have been no shortcuts for her nor me.

Forgiving the unforgivable does not mean forgetting the near-crucifying wounds of colonialism; it does not mean you are weak or disloyal to your culture, and it does not mean you don't seek justice. Forgiving the unforgivable means that you love yourself and life so much that you want to use your energy for what you want to create, rather than spiraling downward because of the past and current pains from what may have happened. Even with all of the horrific past, Maata loves herself and her community so completely that she chooses to do the hard work of forgiving herself and others. Maata focuses completely on using her powerful energy for what she wants to create, a life-giving path forward with the help of her ancestors, nature, community, and culture.

Forgiving the unforgivable is the pathway to freedom, to love of self and others, and it is the passcode to one's own divinity.

If Maata and I were to meet in person, we would share stories of how we experience, firsthand, the deep listening that comes with authentic forgiveness, the patience to allow that forgiveness to emerge without pretense, from the core of being, and how in this patience we feel the presence of the cosmos and ancestors.

I continue to be inspired by Elder Maata's personal stories, leadership, and triumphs over the obstacles created by the ravages of colonialism. Whenever she speaks of these, Maata never fails to emphasize that the path forward is the pursuit of unity in diversity. In this way she is following what her tūpuna, her ancestors, assigned to her as her mission. I can feel her steadfast loyalty to that, her smile, her glow, in my heart. We are joined together for eternity. We will be ancestors together, made kin by our shared vision for this world.

Unity is not only possible; it is necessary.

ANITA SANCHEZ, PH.D., Nahua (Aztec), Toltec, and Mexican American, is committed to bridging Indigenous wisdom with modern science to support leaders, their teams, and businesses to create an environmentally sustainable, spiritually fulfilling, and socially just world. She leads Pachamama Alliance Ecuador Rainforest Journeys deep into the Amazon to live with Indigenous tribes and learn about their deep connection to earth and Indigenous cultures. She is the author of the international, award-winning book *The Four Sacred Gifts: Indigenous Wisdom for Modern Times.*

FOREWORD

A Celebration of Resilience

Jean Hikaka,
daughter of Maata Wharehoka

Tēnā kōutou e te iti e te rahi. He uri ahau nō Ngāti Ranginui, Ngāti Tahinga, Ngāti Apakura, Ngāti Kuia, Ngāti Koata, Ngāti Apa ki te Ra Tō ratou kō Ngāti Toa. Kō Nai Moanaroa tōku koroua. Kō Martha Borrell tōku kuia. Kō Maata tōku māmā. Kō Jean Hikaka tōku ingoa.

I am a descendant of Ngāti Ranginui, Ngāti Tahinga, Ngāti Apakura, Ngāti Kuia, Ngāti Koata, Ngāti Apa ki te Ra Tō ratou kō Ngāti Toa. Nai Moanaroa is my grandfather. Martha Borrell is my grandmother. Maata is my mother. My name is Jean Hikaka.

Oh my gosh, this book has been a labor of love and has needed, at times, huge strength and understanding. The author, Stephania Minesenskji, otherwise known as Stephanie Mines, Ph.D., wanted to write a book to acknowledge and honor our mother Maata Wharehoka (née Moanaroa) with all her pūkenga, and, in doing so, honor all women. This book aims to celebrate resilience, honor the healers, the artists, the wise women, the mothers and grandmothers, the sisters, the dreamers, and the poets. You may find you relate to the many facets of Maata and her journey through life, following her calls from our tūpuna, trusting them always to guide her.

When Stephania arrived in Aotearoa, Mum's health began declining, which meant Mum tired easily. Her stage 4 COPD caused issues, at times giving Stephania a run for her money, with Maata using every kuikui tactic to evade answering questions. It seemed the kūmara (sweet potato) could not talk of its own sweetness. Luckily Mum asked her many friends and whānau to participate by telling their tales of Mum and their encounters, which are now captured in this book.

In the three months Stephania was in Aotearoa, I found her to be respectful, challenging, and wise. She is also super smart. I learned she obtained her Ph.D. in neuroscience while being a single mother. I learned that Stephanie Mines was actually Stephania Minesenskji. Her beautiful Polish/Russian name needed to be changed to fit into Western paradigms. She is also a healer who uses a method called T.A.R.A. (Tools for Awakening Resources and Awareness), and she goes to the gym or exercises daily, keeping herself in tip-top condition. She has a love of people and is very thoughtful and giving.

During the time of the interviews, Mum was seventy-three years old, and Stephania was seventy-nine years old. It was amazing that I was sitting with 152 years of wisdom between them, of which you will now also be able to experience with the sharing of this book.

Stephania has respectfully taken a huge amount of time and effort and resourced the journey to tell Mum's story, a story for all women and a discussion for the world. I hope you may find parts of yourself in the pages or enjoy the wisdom captured or answering the journal questions.

Finally, I leave you with some wisdom my mother always said to me and my brothers and sisters, and now her grandchildren.

> *Be good, if you can't be good, be kind. If you can't be kind, shut your mouth.*
>
> nā Maata Wharehoka

Nāku nā Jean Hikaka is the eldest of Maata's five awesome children. She is passionate about many things, and now that her mother has passed she feels even more passionate about seeing some of her mum's projects through to the end.

Jean trained as a bilingual teacher and while she hasn't taught in a school for almost thirty years, those skills led her to become an educator at Puke Ariki (a heritage site, museum, library, and research center). Jean is also a public health advisor, a Māori health advisor and strategy lead, and a service improvement advisor. She has worked in health for twenty years. Now Jean and her siblings are continuing Maata's business, Kahu Whakatere.

Jean lives at home with her husband Dallas, who is a mental health nurse, and together they have five adult children and thirteen grandchildren.

Entering the Māori Worldview

Indigenous people are our guides to an expansive, welcoming future that will allow our children to flourish. In order for Indigenous wisdom streams to be of service to us, we have to know how to hear them. To absorb traditional insight requires us to shift our worldviews and our ways of relating. This is both corrective and healing. This book helps you walk on a bridge toward unity with all peoples. Fundamental to creating the world we want our children to inherit is the inclusivity and unity that all traditional cultures espouse. As an exponent of this, Maata Wharehoka, the inspiration and central subject of this book, has a vocation of peacemaking. Maata speaks to us from the birthplace of nonviolence, the iconic Parihaka marae, or meeting grounds of the community. She is the living voice of Parihaka's mission of peace.

In these pages we experience Maata's catalyzing influence, love, strength, and creativity as she restores and regenerates Māori culture for her people and the world. She causes us to reflect on how we can ignite our own living experience of belonging and connection. It is only by feeling our kinship with the natural world and with each other that we have any hope of solving the metacrisis conditions that disconnection created. Maata shows us the way.

That way is mapped by the cultivation of cultural sensitivity. This is not just about being polite, or deferential. It is a shift in consciousness and a change of heart. When I first began interviewing Maata and her family and peers, I was an outsider looking in. I was listening and watching. Somewhere, sometime between then and now, I have entered the spaces that I was documenting from the outside. Though I am clearly not Māori by birth, it is as if I have gotten new lenses for my eyes, and I am beginning to see differently, as if from within the world rather than peering at it.

This is why I have included queries at the end of each chapter, inviting readers to take into their lives the places they inhabit and the relationships they have, considerations of cultural sovereignty, and why it is important to stand for values in this world we share. We evolve culture by how we regard and transmit it. If we allow our values to be torn asunder and trashed, then we are party to the disintegration of society and civilization. But if we stand for values that link us to a lineage of values, and evolve those values to adapt to current needs, never losing sight of integrity, then we can claim a legacy worth transmitting.

Maata Wharehoka is the model of holding true to values that come from deeply embodied lineage. She protects those values. The Te Reo Māori word *manaaki* applies here. Manaaki means to protect, to show respect, to take care. The time I have spent at Parihaka, where Maata lives, has infused me with manaaki. The transmission came not only from Maata herself but from the very air, the smells, the harakeke plants, and most of all, the whenua of Parihaka.

As you read this book, as you attune to who Maata is and what Parihaka emanates, and the leadership of Te Whiti o Rongomai and Tohu Kākahi, the originators of nonviolent protest, bear in your mind and heart the spirit of manaaki, the spirit of protection. I invite you to not only respect what is transmitted here but also to protect the values and intentions that I have done my best to relay and that have become part of me as a result of my experience and relationship with Maata Wharehoka and her family.

Entering the Māori worldview is like stepping into a verdant landscape in which humans and plants, animals, the land, the wind, the rain, the mountains, and the rivers, are united, blended, operating from the same intentionality, the same source. This may sound like it is a step into a distant, or even a fantasy, past, but it is actually a view of the future.

Te Ao Māori, the Māori worldview, is wisdom teaching for the world. It will be our salvation to enter the realm where life- and nature-informed consciousness rule every action, every perception, every choice. This is the model of connected living that Maata Wharehoka has been sustaining and regenerating. She is the stamina, the resilience, the adaptability, the inventiveness, and the pragmatic utility of the harakeke. Harakeke is medicinal. It is thick, yet pliable, and by human hands it is woven into clothing, baskets, mats, and art. It can be made so thin that it can be threaded through a needle.

In December 2023, as horrific tragedies continued to unfold after the events of October 7, Maata and I grieved together. Her sense of unity with the suffering of all people comes directly from the lineage of her people and of Te Whiti o Rongomai who predicted that "the nations of the world will be as one." She and I, as mothers and grandmothers, keened for the massacred children, and dedicated ourselves to nonviolence and peace as we sat together in her whare at Parihaka.

I take full responsibility for the errors in this book and for my own ignorance in regard to any misrepresentations or confusion. It is an enormous privilege to be trusted to receive what the Wharehoka family and Maata's friends and peers have shared with me.

It is my intention that this book serves the unity prophesized by Te Whiti o Rongomai. As he was accurate in all his other predictions, I hold on to the accuracy of this one.

Introducing Maata Wharehoka

At the Parihaka marae in the shadow of Mount Taranaki, above the verdant sea cliffs of the North Island of Aotearoa (New Zealand), bordering the Tasman Sea, the thick fronds of the harakeke clap in the gusty wind like an audience applauding. The bright coral ngutukaka flowers, the pristine mānuka blossoms and kōkohurangi (tree daisies) dance around the harakeke, as if they were children, bowing to a queen mother.

At the top of a winding road, surrounded by pasture meadows and nearly forty-five kilometers from New Plymouth, the nearest Pākehā town and regional center is Maata's home. Like the harakeke outside her door, she reigns there, and her mokopuna (grandchildren) along with her daughters and sons, are her mānuka blossoms. Maata has the fortitude, the sturdiness, and the intention to serve her people that is just like the hardy harakeke, also native to Aotearoa, and of which she is a master weaver.

The rooms and walls of her whare (home) hold all the chapters in the compelling saga of Maata's tireless devotion to her whānau (family), to Te Ao Māori (the Māori world view) and to Parihaka, about which you will hear a great deal in this book. When you enter the house, the first room is the spacious lounge, the wharenui, often filled with the play of children. The kitchen is the belly of the house, where food is shared generously with all who enter, including visitors, volunteers, interviewers like me, and community members.

And then there is Maata's room, the place where she rests, sleeps, reads, writes, creates art, and where Kahu Whakatere, the rite of passage for death and dying, was reborn. This is the room where Maata's sister Millie and Maata's husband, Te Ru, died, and through their deaths, contributed to the emergence of the cultural reclamation that is Kahu Whakatere. An entire chapter in this book is devoted to this because Kahu Whakatere encompasses every aspect of Maata's legacy.

In the days of the third and final cycle of her life, Maata Wharehoka, despite illness and pain, is filled with the dynamic resilience of spirit, the life force or mana that was obvious to others in her childhood and her youth, indeed throughout her life, and that radiates from her even now.

Maata was not born in Parihaka, but she will die there, in that same room where her sister and husband died, wrapped in garments woven of harakeke. Her body will be at ease on a soft mat, still redolent with the earthy, fresh scent of the plants from which it was made, and woven by her family and her community. Her tenacious body, with all its accumulated struggles and burdens, its memories of mischief and defiance, of love and rebellion, will let go and be received into the land that is her source, her identity. She will be welcomed into the cool, protective shade of her mountain, Taranaki.

Like the women she most emulates and reveres, Te Puea and Eva Rickard, Maata is multigifted, multiskilled. Consider how these women would have lived and contributed to their communities without the racism and colonialism that shaped their expression. They are artists, community organizers, healthcare providers, mothers, grandmothers, prophets, and innovators. They are voices for the living earth from which they feel no separation. They emanate from the land and the people they adore. Maata Wharehoka draws from their modeling and Maata's life will instill this lineage in all the young Māori women seeking it.

Maata's youthful countenance projects and transmits the primordial fire of her spirit, her mauri. Her bright face belies the suffering from illnesses that have plagued her for decades. The cords of her oxygen machine trail her wherever she goes. Her pain spasms are marked by a sudden silence and the closing of her eyes; a brief pause in her relentless extensions outward to fulfill her destiny. She keeps these interludes of unbearable pain to herself; she endures them internally, and then resumes her weaving or her transmission to her moko (diminutive for mokopuna or grandchildren) or one of her adult children, whoever is available. Everyone honors her choice now to just be with the pain. They accompany her in her silence. In these moments we pray together to ease her suffering.

Maata arrived in Taranaki in 1981 to work as a nurse at the Base Hospital in New Plymouth. On her first visit to Parihaka as part of a nurse's group, she felt an immediate connection to its history. It was there that she was introduced to Te Ru, and by 1987 they had established themselves as a family. Maata wanted her daughter Puna to be the first baby born on the marae in a long time, and while circumstances prevented that occurrence exactly as Maata would have preferred, Puna was still a child born of Parihaka, the first offspring of Maata and Te Ru. "After decades of desolation," Maata says, "her birth set the benchmark for families to follow."

Later offspring Ngahina and Te Akau joined their sister, and Maata's two children from previous relationships, Jean and Elias. The Wharehoka's were, in those early days, a new united front of leadership, optimism, and regeneration for Parihaka. This whānau (family) remains an indestructible united front, and Te Ru, known fondly as Papa, though deceased, will always be a vital presence.

When Maata passes, her imprint will remain. Each member of this family will inherit a portion of the mantle that Maata refers to as her destiny, her purpose in being as a human, as a woman, as Māori.

The tower of feminine leadership that is Maata Wharehoka came from humble origins, in rural Tauranga. Her family's tribal affiliations connect her with renowned Kuia Te Puea and Eva Rickard. Raised with deep respect for Te Ao Māori, the Māori worldview, Maata rises like a phoenix from the ashes of the time when Te Reo, the Māori language, was forbidden, and tikanga, Māori traditional practices, were suppressed. Every action Maata takes, every word she speaks, is for the reclamation of her cultural sovereignty.

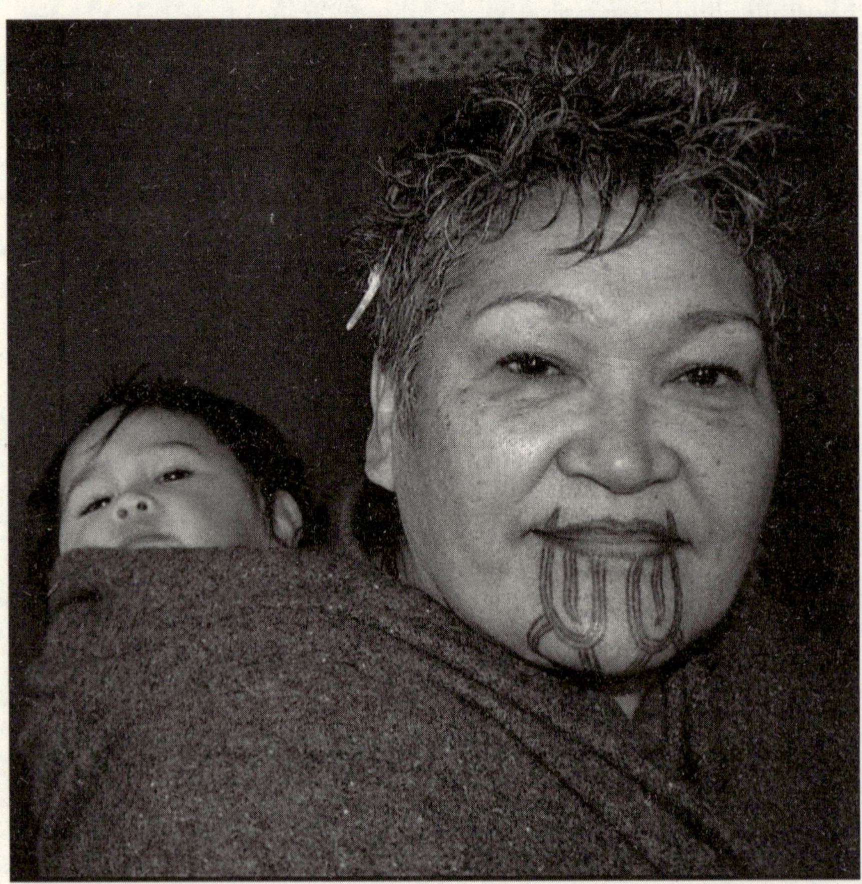

She transmits this with feminine confidence, through her presence, her art, her poetry, and her bearing. In this way she is a treasure to young Māori women and girls, as you will read in these pages, and to women everywhere who have been disconnected from who they truly are. This is why the women who meet her, whether or not they are Māori, want to sit at her feet and just listen to her, hear her stories, and be part of her unflappable, focused aura.

The dignity that is innate in Maata, combined with her straightforward manner, her ability to orchestrate events and connect people, and her diverse artistry, has been, beginning at a young age, a harbinger of a postcolonial era of leadership for Māori women at a time of global transition. Long before the #MeToo movement, Maata advocated for women's rights. This is one of many illustrations of her prophetic nature and why her legacy needs to be transmitted beyond Aotearoa.

Maata Wharehoka is harakeke, the flax fiber plant that is native to Aotearoa. The many strands of the harakeke plants, which grow in abundance around Maata's home, are symbolic of the variegated fibers within Maata herself. Every strand of who she is has been braided into her personal and collective whānau (family) and Te Ao Māori. As a woman, a mother, a grandmother, and a great-grandmother, as the matriarch of Parihaka, Maata Wharehoka has the stamina, the adaptability, the resilience, and the multifaceted functioning of the harakeke. She is like the outside leaves of the plant that serve to protect the inner shoots and the smaller leaves that are the offspring of the awhi rito (parent leaves).

Plants like harakeke give rise to inventiveness. Māori weavers, such as Maata, utilize harakeke for an assortment of purposes. The fiber is for weaving clothing, works of art, and containers, like baskets. The sap is medicinal. The strands are so strong they can hold even the heaviest things, and so fine that they can be threaded into

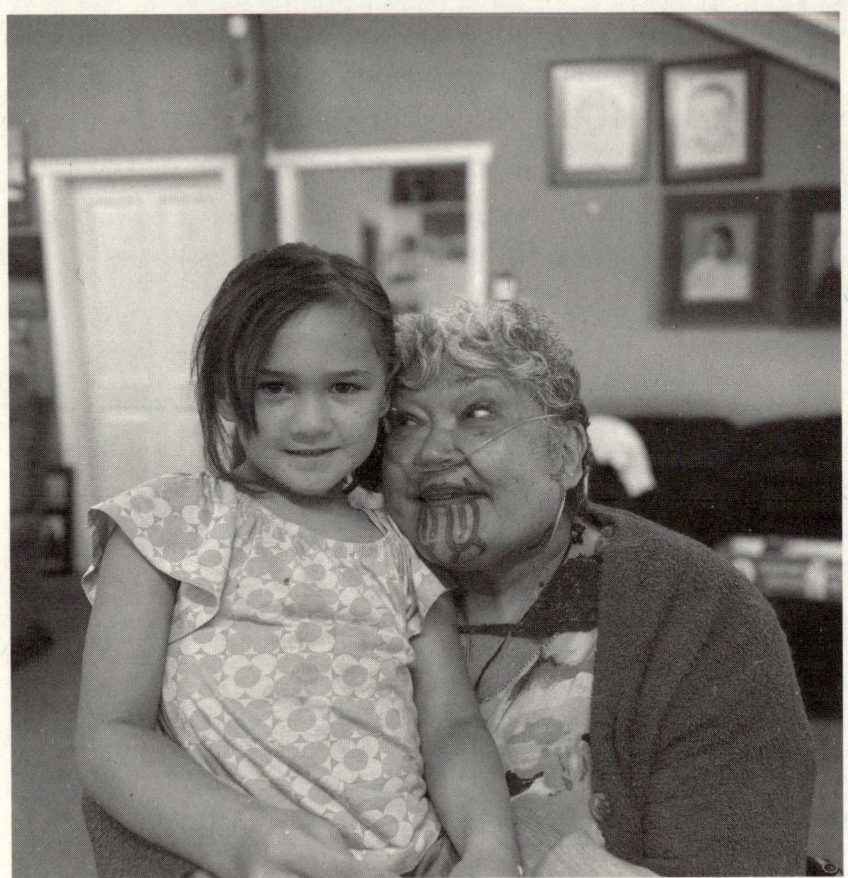

a sewing needle. The long fibers of the plant need to be softened if they are to be used in weaving. This can be done by hand, but Maata designed a machine that softens the strands so that the threads become malleable. This is what I mean when I say that Maata sustains and regenerates Te Ao Māori.

Maata restores precolonial leadership roles for women by her actions and presence. It is only the patriarchal theft of women's voices that has distorted how we perceive women in Aotearoa, and everywhere in the world. What Maata Wharehoka embodies is women's innate authority and vibrance. This is the inheritance of all women.

1

Belonging

You inhabit me. I inhabit you.

Stan Walker

Belonging is inscribed in Māoridom. In contrast, dominant cultural forces are splintering, separating, fragmenting, and polarizing. They try to pry us apart from one another, and from ourselves. What can we learn from Māori about the innate belonging that defies hegemony? This chapter spells out this transmission, and how Maata Wharehoka, and women like her, embody it.

In reclaiming their belonging despite the devastating wounds inflicted on them by colonizers, the tangata whenua, the people of the land, offer us a model to alchemize the disinheritance weaponized by colonization. The death throes of modernity and concomitant metacrisis insist that we pay attention to the teachings of Indigenous peoples. Considering how assiduously Pākehā (Europeans) apply themselves to dismantling the integrity of Māori people and their cultural institutions, it is miraculous that the inherent sense of belonging integral to Māori family systems and collective consciousness is so vital now and steadily gaining momentum.

Let's look respectfully at Māori methodologies of restoration, as demonstrated by and through people like Maata Wharehoka.

Maata was once Carol, and her husband Te Ru, was once Richard. Reclaiming their true names began a new chapter in their personal and collective lives. In the spirit of belonging, their leadership is, and always will be, for their people. As Maata said to me, "It has never occurred to me that I am leading. Rather, I have been led. I am leading according to mandate."

For Maata, inclusivity and belonging go hand in hand. Her motivations for truth and reconciliation are never vengeful. Rather, they are borne out of rootedness. Belonging is not ownership. It is relationship. It is because of her relationship to everyone and everything that Maata Wharehoka emanates and conveys the essence of belonging. To be steadfast in this relationship, even though Pākehā make every attempt, with considerable force, to uproot it, is the founding principle of the reclamation of sovereignty. Perseverance, with unquestionable confidence, is what we are called to decipher and emulate. When Maata Wharehoka clarified her mandate for herself, through the transmission of her tūpuna (ancestors), there was no stopping her, no turning back. Maata is discernment; her eye never wavers from her goal for her people, and thereby for all people. They are one and the same. Conveying this intentionality, and imparting it as accessible, realizable, practical, and essential is the message and purpose of this book.

Maata spent decades moving through rage, grief, loss, and insult. That these fissures have been repaired is to her tribute and the tribute of her tūpuna. Whenua, as you will be reminded often in these pages, is also the Te Reo Māori word for placenta, the nourishing organ of the womb. This tells you how tortuous it was for Māori to have their land stolen from them. It was the same as if their babies were robbed of their nourishing placentas and left to starve and die, unprotected. In the end, though, this theft only deepened their sense of belonging.

Imagine the humiliation and outrage when Māori are required to buy their own land, or pay rent to live on it? As Maata Wharehoka says in her poem "Emancipation," quoted here with her consent, only spiritual fortitude has overcome these insults and violations.

Our people are marginalized,
Their land taken away,
To be able to live a life now,
For everything they must pay.
So why do we carry on?
We do so to keep our spirit alive.
When we see the truth
We know we will survive.

Maata knows the Pākehā world from the inside. She has, you might say, dual citizenship. She was instilled with Pākehā values and mores by an aunt with whom she lived during her formative years; she attended Pākehā institutions of learning, and her first marriage was to a Pākehā man. After having experienced that other world, though, Maata has chosen to dedicate herself to her Māori roots and to beckon other Māori home to where their sense of belonging feeds them—where they are, to use Maata's word, "homegrown." Similarly, Maata chose the path of advocating for her people over other potential vocations. She is not the only one; Acclaimed Māori writer Patricia Grace (2021, 18), who also could have been fragmented by the diverse cultures she inhabited, speaks to this from her experience.

> I grew up amid two worlds, having close, continuous, and frequent contact with each. These were two different and contrasting

spheres that I inhabited, both full of life and vitality: my mother's Pākehā family and my father's Māori whānau.

This statement is made early in Patrica Grace's memoir, *From the Centre: A Writer's Life*. It reflects her strong sense of belonging to a place, Aotearoa, to all her people, and to herself. Later in life, when Patricia Grace invested herself in restoring the marae on her people's land, and when she, against the recommendation of others, said that she would use Te Reo in her writing, without any explanation to Pākehā readers, she declared her allegiances. "I have made up my mind," she said, speaking from the core of her confidence. This is belonging.

The Journey to Belonging

> *Māori women's stories have been relegated to the margins of history. There are things that we don't know about ourselves because the stories about who we are have been censored and omitted from the record.*
>
> Ngāhuia Murphy

Long before the concepts of feminism reached Aotearoa, Maata Wharehoka was an oracle of women's empowerment. Her voice must be included in the resounding, and growing, chorus for our living earth via women's transdisciplinary, outspoken leadership. Maata deserves a place alongside her global sisters. Women like Maya Angelou, Dolores Huerta, Joy Harjo, Robin Wall Kimmerer, Bella Abzug, Rigoberta Menchu, Wangari Maathai, and Ellen Johnson Sirleaf would embrace her as one of their own if they knew of her and met her. I consider this book an introduction to them, whether on the earth plane or beyond, to welcome her into their circle. Like these women, who celebrate and embody belonging as a feminine principle, Maata's journey is demanding, and sometimes excruciating. Her near-death experiences are landmarks, each one amplifying the sustaining, nutritive power of belonging.

When Maata's son, Te Akau Wharehoka, says that his mother "knows what it is like to be Pākehā; she knows what it is like to be Pasifika, and she knows what it is to be Māori," he is referring to Maata's experiences in her marriages to a Pākehā man, a Pasifika man, and then to Te Ru Wharehoka, Te Akau's father. The Pākehā and Pasifika marriages were rites of passage that challenged and sometimes threatened the well-being of Maata and her family. This is not an uncommon rite of passage for women leaders. The memoirs of Maya Angelou and Joy Harjo, for instance, report on the obstacle courses that women, through their relationships and partnerships, surmount on the path to self-manifestation.

Belonging may be the most precious gift Maata delivers to every Māori wahine (female), and to every Māori whānau (family) that she encounters. It is the treasure she has claimed for herself through her chosen name, her chosen language, and with every hard-earned breath she takes.

The Toll of Family Violence on Belonging

Violence and fragmentation are the insignias of colonization. Violence binds victim and perpetrator in a fatalistic pas de deux. Unraveling these overcoupled choreographies requires profound cultural knowledge. New Zealand has very high rates of family violence among all ethnic groups, but Māori rates are highest. Presettlement and precolonization, Māori society addressed family violence using traditional songs and stories, conveyed in healing circles that referenced the creation tales known to every community member. The reverberations of interpersonal abuse, whether physical, psychological, emotional, spiritual, or sexual, were always felt, held, and acknowledged by the collective in traditional Māori communities. It was also the collective, the regional group, and the tribe, from which flowed the methodologies of reconciliation, recovery, remorse, and compensation. As Māori researcher and scholar Denise Wilson (2023, 2) points out, "When addressing prevention and healing, victim and perpetrator terminology is unhelpful for achieving solutions."

In the creation story of Papatūānuku and Ranginui (earth and heaven, respectively), the original family struggles, parents and offspring fighting against each other, in the movement from darkness to light. The forces of the natural world became engaged in the fractious reorganization of the family structure and participated through furious actions aimed to restore unity, but never fully succeeded. Ultimately it is the profound, indestructible love of Papa (mother) and Rangi (father) that sustains everyone and everything. My retelling here is a simplification of much more complex stories and substories in the intricate and exquisite mythology of the creation of the world and human beings. The key message for this chapter is that disputes are inevitable and all aspects of the environment cohere to find resolution. The entire world holds us in love as we seek to know the truth of what unites us.

It is her deep love for her people, like Papatūānuku's love for her children that was so strong she refused to be separated from them, that urges Maata to be available to offer her wisdom and knowledge of tikanga (Māori practices) for families experiencing abuse. Her strong presence is a refuge. She walks her talk. She knows the full scope of what families endure, and she knows the origins of their suffering. I was privileged to be with her as she invited young women to partake of her strength and to find sanctuary in her presence. On the sacred grounds of Parihaka, or anywhere else she was, I have seen Maata offer the space beside her, patting it gently and invitingly with her strong, hard-working hand, to young women longing for a role model they can trust.

Maata awakens every Māori woman's innate memory of the presettler power they used to have and shows them that they can embody that now. She reminds those she counsels of when Māori women had authority and status and thus encourages them to claim that which is theirs. Colonization stole this inheritance from Māori women by marginalizing them, but Maata restores it with her every word and every action on behalf of her people.

Māori women experiencing violence in their homes are bereft of their relationship to themselves as well as to their culture, and they are excruciatingly conscious of the impacts of violence on their families. Maata clarifies for them, and for everyone really, whether Māori or not, just as she has clarified for herself, that the first step toward safety is cultural belonging, and that this belonging can only be known somatically. It cannot be dictated.

Violent re-enactment is the dark side of a love that has been distorted, twisted, traumatized, and contorted. The unwinding, Maata discovered, is ignited by connection, by true, unquestionable belonging and cultural sovereignty. That is what unravels the convoluted impulses that are the by-product of separation and disinheritance. As the tall, outer leaves of the harakeke grow higher and thicker to protect the innocent, small harakeke babies in the center of the plant, so does Maata lead Māori back home to their prophetic culture, at the heart of which are the children, the tamariki.

Moko Kauwae Is Not Just a Tattoo

My moko kauwae was the beginning of my journey in being strong as a Māori woman. Even though my skin is white, the way that I am is Māori. I have a heart-to-heart connection with my tūpuna. My moko kauwae was guided by them.

JEAN HIKAKA

The tapping of the poi (colorful balls at the end of strings swung in rhythm to music, song, and dance); the chants and prayers intoned by the kuia (female elders); the rain outside just as the ceremony began, these were the analgesics for Jean, Maata's eldest daughter, at her moko papa ceremony where she received the moko kauwae or chin tattoo. For Māori women, this is the insignia of belonging and utter confidence in their Māori identity. Women experience moko papa only after deep reflection on their relationship to Te Ao Māori.

The moko kauwae originates in a myth that tells of Mataora, whose name means *the living face.* He brought the art of moko up from the underworld. The story is told that Mataora abused his wife, Niwareka, and she fled from his violence. He pursued her, begging for forgiveness. With the help of Uetonga, Niwareka's father, they were reconciled. Uetonga then taught Mataora the art of tā moko, by making him the first one to endure the pain of receiving it.

Being Māori is much more than appearances. Even in speaking Te Reo, language is not only the use of the words. It is the intention behind the words. Just having Te Reo is not enough. Getting the moko is similar, whether for men or women. In all things Māori, everything is about connection with tūpuna, with ancestors. Moko is not just a tattoo. It is the reflection of an inner state of being.

> *Taia o moko, hai hoa matenga mou.*
> *Of your moko, you cannot be deprived, except*
> *by death.*
> *It will be your ornament, and your companion,*
> *until your last day.*
>
> Māori Proverb

The reclamation of tā moko (the art of the Māori tattoo) is the inscription of identity. Dermographic art is a visible proclamation of selfhood. It speaks of one's kinship: a testimony of devotion to community. Tā moko is the intricate, expressed, and demonstrable allegiance with what it means to be Māori, and of the connection Māori always have to their ancestors.

The reclamation of Te Reo and tā moko speaks to current and future Māori about what it means to liberate oneself from the ramifications of colonization and conscription. The Māori population plummeted by as much as 60 percent over the late nineteenth and early twentieth centuries because of the introduction of lethal diseases. High infant mortality proceeded into the 1950s. Now, as the Māori population regains vitality and steadily increases, and as traditional rites of passage return the truth of Māori culture to children and youth, the symbols of belonging, like tā moko, speak volumes. Maata's choice to receive her moko kauwae as a mature woman rediscovering her Māori roots sends a strong, clear message to young people who face a future of mounting insecurities. Maata weaves the tapestry from the past, through the present, and into a future that we cannot predict, but which is woven with the sturdy fibers of belonging.

The Marae Is Tūrangawaewae: A Place to Stand

It is stunning to note that some of Aotearoa's most stalwart and effective women leaders have invested themselves in reconstructing, building, or creating marae for their people. Here is what Dame Iritana Tawhiwhirangi (1992), a Māori language champion, says about the marae: "The marae has endured for generations. It is a place of key significance. It is sustained by and for families. Marae are the caretakers of whānau. Marae revitalizes the spirit of a people."

Women like Te Puea, Maata Wharehoka, and Patricia Grace have poured their life energies into establishing centers where the community can come together, share experiences, raise children, and nurture land and connection. The traditional marae is the manifestation of the whenua, the placenta, the womb of life for tangata whenua. The marae is more than a place. Like tā moko, it is a state of consciousness.

It is on the marae that younger generations learn directly from their family members and elders. Many marae require reconstruction, or must be built from the ground up, after their sites were ravaged and desecrated by settlers. The world knows very little about the hard-working Māori women of Aotearoa who regenerated marae. When Maata and her husband Te Ru returned to Parihaka, it was a ghost town. They revitalized the epic site that was of such enormous value to Māori and the entire world. Please read more about Parihaka, and Maata's commitment to its revitalization, in the chapter in this book dedicated to it.

What do we learn about women and belonging from Te Puea, Patricia Grace, and Maata about the role of the collective, the gathering together of people in kinship with their focused solidarity on sacred land? Is it not utterly feminine to devote oneself to creating such a place? Just as women are the whare (home) of the tangata (people), so are they the ones who know the enduring, life-giving power of containing, nurturing, and educating them about who they really are and who imparts the birthright of belonging.

Te Puea Herangi, who Maata greatly admired and who was a role model for her, advocated for and invested her mana (life force) to build the marae called *Tūrangawaewae*, which means a place to stand. Against all odds, Te Puea built not only a marae, she also created a thriving farm, a sanctuary for orphans, and a clinic where healthcare for Māori was provided by Māori, in a location where they would feel comfortable. This healthcare model was exceptionally meaningful to Maata, when as a public health nurse, she saw that Māori women were disrespected in cervical cancer screenings and therefore did not comply. Maata revolutionized the system with culturally sensitive healthcare, inspired by Te Puea.

Tūrangawaewae became the base from which Te Puea could advocate for Māori sovereignty and autonomy, and launch campaigns for reparations for stolen land. She supported and encouraged Māori leadership, resulting in some of her protégés becoming members of Parliament, and then endorsing her initiatives. As her destiny directed her, Te Puea became more and more effective in legislative circles without ever losing sight of her humility and priorities.

Tūrangawaewae was securely established by the mid-1930s. It was a home for those who had been stripped of their land, it was an educational center, and a source of economic freedom through the farm industries Te Puea initiated. Tūrangawaewae was also, if not primarily, a place for young people, many of whom were orphaned by the ravaging influenza outbreaks and illnesses imported by Europeans. Te Puea gathered them together and gave them a home and a family. Tūrangawaewae was a place of unity. Te Puea was a model for Maata in developing functional, friendly partnerships with Pākehā, while maintaining Māori traditions in daily practice so that all Māori knew who they were and where they were rooted. Maata Wharehoka has been masterful with this kind of multicultural networking, inspired by Te Puea.

Patricia Grace, one of New Zealand's foremost literary figures, devoted herself to building the marae, with her husband and her community, in Hongoeka Bay. This devotion required learning the weaving and carving that would make it possible for the structures to be a repository of Ngāti Toa history. While writing award-winning books and raising her family, Patricia Grace joined with her iwi (tribe) and hapū (regional group) to construct buildings and courtyards from the ground up. The trees from which the beams of the buildings were made were seen as wombs, and the carvings done according to guidance from masters who knew that they were creating art as well as structures for the people to use. Each master of carving or weaving who was involved consciously imparted their life force, and the blessings of their ancestors, into the structures, all for their tamariki, the children of the future.

After years of hard work, the marae was opened with a commemoration ceremony, in 1997. Now there was a place for the children to learn their history, their language, to celebrate their holidays, to hold social events, and to mourn the dead, according to their traditions. It was even the place where the All Blacks came in 2017 to learn a Ngāti Toa haka for the World Cup. The haka was a celebration of life, written by a tūpuna (elder) in 1820, when he was able to escape soldiers determined to kill him, because of the sanctuary that he received from the Ngāti Toa people who hid him from the troops.

Tariana Turia, who was responsible for the birth of the Māori Party, also devoted herself to the establishment of a marae that would be a refuge for youth. Te Awa, housed on the marae that

Tariana and her husband rebuilt in Whangaehu, became a bustling village for young people.

In addition to being a member of Parliament, Tariana Turia never wavered from her commitment to her marae, to the health of her people, and to the upliftment of youth. She campaigned vociferously to stop the tobacco industry from toxically manipulating her people. Maata did the same by insisting that tobacco not be used in the meeting halls of Parihaka. Her kuia law is respected to this day. Both Maata and Tariana campaigned for services for youth. Both of them personally fostered youth whenever they could, giving them a place to call home on the marae that they themselves were instrumental in rebuilding, with their own hands.

Maata Wharehoka's granddaughter, Hotukura, speaks of the developmental importance of the marae.

> Our wharenui (meeting-house), Te Niho o te Atiawa, is a house that shelters, protects, and binds me to my Taranaki roots. . . . I spent much of my childhood at Parihaka and at various hui (meetings) throughout the rohe (district). My grandparents worked hard, alongside others, to rebuild Te Niho o te Atiawa and to demand the return of our whenua (land). . . . Taranaki is a coastal and mountainous region on the western side of Te Ika a Māui (the North Island) of Aotearoa (New Zealand). Parihaka is a Māori settlement located halfway between the base of Taranaki mounga (mountain) and the west coast of Te Ika a Māui, the North Island of Aotearoa/New Zealand. I remember playing on the old concrete foundations of Te Raukura, climbing the hills and wandering in the gorse. However, I was forced to sit still sometimes, and it was during those times that I heard our stories, observed our protocols, and watched my elders perform their respective roles. It is to the sound of many waiata (songs) that I

> fell asleep, or clumsily flailed my poi. . . . The sound of those poi beating is just as etched in, and on, my body as the beating of my own heart (Seed-Pihama, 2017, 1–2).

Maata and her husband Te Ru worked diligently, along with other families, to restore Parihaka to its epic status, when they married and moved back to the marae with Maata's children, Jean and Elias. Puna, Ngahina, and Te Akau were conceived and raised at Parihaka. They grew up speaking Te Reo as their first language. Their lives embody the restoration of Parihaka. Te Akau is a contractor and is, as I write this, rebuilding the dining hall and kitchen for Te Niho. Dining halls and kitchens are the bellies of the marae. I experienced turning-point moments in the old dining hall at Te Niho, amid the lively chatter and smiles of the Parihaka community. These events, organized by the avidly community-minded Maata Wharehoka, were designed by her in her prophetic wisdom and in the lineage of Te Whiti and Tohu, to bring people together so that the mystery of life could unfold. Thanks to Maata's work these buildings where people gather throughout Parihaka are designated as no-smoking structures, assuring that they are welcoming and safe for all.

Belonging Beyond Time and Space

What differentiates the Māori concept of lineage and belonging from the Western, dominant culture definition is that Māori are connected to the beginning of time and to all aspects of the environment. Humans, Te Ao Māori says, are interdependent with ecosystems, and, in the end, everyone is descended from the same lineage. Westerners would do well to consider this as an antidote to the epidemics of loneliness, alienation, anxiety, and polarization that are afflicting humanity. The knowledge of kinship that transcends time and space is cellular, and while Europeans shrouded and obfuscated that wisdom for a time, they are no longer able to do that. The truth is on the rise, and it is contagious.

Maata Wharehoka belongs to herself. This is the same as saying that she belongs to her tūpuna and that she belongs to the forces of creation that made her the voice of her people. In her silence, as pain moves through her body, she is with her tūpuna. In her belonging that is beyond time and space, she listens to them. Her tūpuna are guiding her. Maata is having those conversations even as I write these words. She is crossing over, moving beyond time and space. She knows, as the title of a poem she wrote states, that "this is not the end."

REFLECTIONS ON BELONGING

1. Have you ever been betrayed? How did you recover from this, and how did you find your way back to wholeness, if you have? If you have not, what is missing? What makes it possible to come out of the shattering and fragmentation of betrayal? How is it possible to find wholeness and trust again? Through this exploration of yourself, you will have a sense of the healing that Māori have done and are doing in order to move forward in and with the world.
2. What expression of your cultural identity is sacred to you? If there is nothing that you can reference in response to this inquiry, create an imaginary act, ritual, or behavior that could allow you to experience the sacred nature of belonging. Describe it here. Provide photos, drawings, and any art that communicates your discovery of sacred belonging.
3. If you could invent a symbolic representation of how you honor and feel connected to your cultural identity, what would that be? Do not feel limited by words; feel free to use art, sound, music, movement, or any other form of expression. Think of

the Palestinian scarf and the Jewish yarmulke. It takes courage to present your cultural identity in such an outward-facing manner. Do you want to do that, or would you prefer to be more private about your cultural identity? Explain.

4. What is your feeling when you see tā moko on Māori people? Be honest. Do you feel aesthetic appreciation? Fear? Curiosity? Anything else? Would you choose such a rite of passage as receiving tā moko and its unerasable statement of identity? Whether your answer is yes or no, please explain.
5. Do you have a tūrangawaewae, a place to stand? Where is it? How often do you stand there? What happens when you do? Who shares that space with you?
6. How do you express your experience of being part of a human collective, of being a member of humanity, with dignity and love?
7. If everything you did was intended to serve future generations, how would that change how you orient your life?
8. Are you inspired, daunted, or discouraged by the concept that you have a responsibility to future generations? Explain.
9. What do you create that could be considered similar to tā moko or to other traditional arts? If there is nothing yet in your life like this, have you considered what you could commit to doing like this to honor your legacy?
10. Do you come from a background of different cultures, like Patricia Grace, the Māori writer whose quote about her Māori father and Pākehā mother appears in this chapter? If yes, what impact does this have on your sense of belonging? Tell the story of how you found your own identity and sense of belonging from and with your cultural background, which most likely has multicultural origins. If you have not yet written this story, consider writing it and sharing it with others. What, if anything, has held you back from doing this before?

2

Parihaka

He kakano i ruia mai i Rangiatea.
The seed will not be lost.

MĀORI PROVERB

Redeeming Peace

Maata lives, and will die, on the land where Māori staked their claim for truth and never gave up. As the lyrics to the song "Parihaka" by Tim Finn say: "I'll sing to you the song of Parihaka. The spirit of nonviolence has come to fill the silence."

The song narrates the tale of Te Whiti o Rongomai, the most well-known of those who were the original strategists of nonviolent resistance to tyranny, rape, and devastation, on the very land where Maata Wharehoka and her family now abide as caretakers.

The papakāinga, original home base, of Parihaka, with all its dwellings and gardens, is arranged like a crinoline underskirt, spread out along the western foothills of Mount Taranaki. "Te Whiti o Rongomai was asked to describe what happened at Parihaka on November 5, 1881, when fifteen hundred armed soldiers arrived to plunder the land of the Māori, to rape the women, and massacre the innocent, unarmed people, including children. His response was recorded by historian Dick Scott in his book *Ask That Mountain*, which is dedicated to the uncle of Te Ru Wharehoka, Maata's husband: "The white man in his covetousness ordered me to move on instead of removing himself from my land. I resisted. I resist to this day." At this point, Scott (2006, 1) reports that Te Whiti pointed to the mountain. "Ask that mountain," he said. "Taranaki saw it all."

Humble, unpretentious, simple, and yet mythic at the same time, Parihaka is a labyrinth of small and medium-sized dwellings, winding dirt roads, meeting houses, an award-winning sprawling community garden overflowing with vegetables, lettuces, gourds, kūmara, and a wealth of herbs. It wasn't long after her arrival in Taranaki in 1981 that Maata Wharehoka went to Parihaka, with a group of Māori nurses. "I felt an immediate connection," she reflected, later. The timeless, sacred, and momentous nature of Parihaka is immediately tangible. You know, as soon as you set foot on the land, that you are walking where history has been made; where a holy teaching resides. Your voice softens, and for some, like me, tears well up, and then fall profusely, even before a word is uttered.

This is the place where the concepts and logistics of Mahatma Gandhi and Dr. Martin Luther King Jr. originated. Their descendants went to Parihaka in 2005 to pay homage at the urupā (cemetery) where Te Whiti and Tohu are buried and to touch the ground where plowshares defied guns, swords, and rapacious greed. Though hardly known, the story of Parihaka is a compelling narrative for this moment in time. Its teachings speak directly to the struggles now tearing humanity and civilization to shreds. One of the purposes of this book is to propagate Parihaka's pedagogy, which Maata Wharehoka has consistently maintained and evolved. She, along with others, has been instrumental in reviving the Parihaka papakāinga and reactivating its intended spirit of education, unity, hospitality, and triumph over the odds. Her legacy speaks to us from Parihaka, in the soft or tumultuous winds, in the hushed, awed sense of people engaged in traditional practices that they learn from elders like Maata, and in the narratives that are on the tip of her tongue and that relay the resurrection and prophetic guidance of Parihaka.

It took over one hundred years for the Crown, the British colonial system, to apologize for its actions at Parihaka. In 2017, Chris Finlayson, Treaty Negotiations Minister, came to Parihaka to deliver an expression of remorse. Just as invading soldiers in 1881 were met by offerings of food and song, so was Finlayson greeted with hospitality, despite the unabashed flow of tears on all sides. It took two more years after that for the apology to become law in the form of the Parihaka Reconciliation Bill.

Yes. Parihaka is an epic landmark site in world history, but it is also Maata Wharehoka's home. It is where her grandchildren do their homework. It is where relatives come to visit and holidays are celebrated. It is where songs are sung and art is made. It is where Maata, a matriarch of the place, holds court. Whether from her bed where she is resting from a bout of pain, or from a comfy, cushy couch in the big lounge, or from around the kitchen table, Maata is unquestionably a rangatira, the authority. When you enter her whare (home), the first place you go to is wherever Maata is.

As she walks from room to room, her oxygen cords trailing her like life-giving minions, or when she goes outside to harvest harakeke, pushing her walker or riding in her automated wheelchair with its basket of collected herbs, scissors, clothes, and tools, Maata is like an empress of Parihaka. Her crown is made of the feathers that adorn her hair and that are somehow always secure on her head, regardless of the weather. These feathers remind us that her eye is always on the sparrow, always on the goals of ending racism and restoring justice, and that these goals are firm, regardless of the circumstances.

Te Whiti o Rongomai, the prescient, charismatic orator, the embodiment of nonviolent resistance and the strategist, along with his uncle, Tohu Kākahi, the second arm of Parihaka's leadership, made their homes and lived out their lives at Parihaka. Reviled and feared by the Pākehā settlers, Te Whiti and Tohu followed deep spiritual guidance. It was to the God of the New Testament that Te Whiti and Tohu prayed. They prayed for the very people who had given them that Bible, but who acted as if they had never read it.

There is no formal church at Parihaka. The meeting houses, like Te Niho, where Maata is the kaitiaki (caretaker/guardian), serve like churches in terms of community gathering and education, storytelling (kōrero), and transmission. Maata calls it the "meeting house to all the students of the world." "This," she says, "is how this house is managed." I have had the good fortune to be in Te Niho when Maata is making her networking magic, bringing people together, generating evocative, emergent conversations, and making sure that sumptuous, celebratory meals are shared, the clatter of plates matching the active voices of all present.

It is from Te Niho that Maata fulfills Te Whiti's instructions that people from everywhere in the world come there to learn about peacemaking. Maata is the organizer of those instructive gatherings, seeing to every detail, networking to bring thousands and thousands of people to Parihaka, never forgetting Te Whiti's legacy. It is at Te Niho where visitors can feel, from the very first moment that they are there, the swell of hope that came when Māori first congregated to consider their future, first shared kōrero (dialogues) with one another about their fears for their children, and listened to the wisdom and forecasts of Te Whiti and Tohu, who never let them down and who were always accurate. Maata restores the same deep listening that was embodied at that time, the same prophetic, visionary conceptualizing that was the hallmark of Te Whiti and Tohu, and the same quality of calls to action that serve the people by voicing their truth for and with them.

The early residents of Parihaka made a collective choice to engage in the risky experiment of nonviolent resistance. The settlers assumed that they could easily defeat the Māori people. Pākehā still make this assumption. They were wrong then, and they are wrong now. The Māori population is growing in Aotearoa. They have not died out as predicted. In fact, Māori culture is in the full thrust of a cultural renaissance that just keeps expanding. Maata Wharehoka is one of the vibrant leaders of that renaissance. She, along with other elders, is restoring the beauty and dignity of Kaupapa Māori. Maata is resolute and staunch in maintaining tikanga practices to ensure the continuity of culture, cultural practices, and cultural sovereignty.

While projecting onto Māori that they were inferior and ignorant, the settlers robbed them of their farms and homelands. They implanted the seeds of massive, splintering psychological warfare, coupled with crimes of inhumanity, sexual abuse, and torture. The strategies were ruthless and aimed at genocide. If we take the long view, the settlers failed. But they did inflict enormous, long-lasting suffering. The healing will take lifetimes, but it is happening apace, and it will continue.

Parihaka is where no one is forgotten. The children are still singing, and the women are still baking bread, just as they did on the day the settlers arrived. The atmosphere is redolent with unconditional love, rising from the moist, fertile earth that has never ceased to feed the tangata whenua, the people of the land. Deep purple and delicately hued lavender-colored teiria (dahlias) cluster like flamboyant family groupings, full of life and promise. Parihaka is the place of redemption and resurgence. Freedom is in the air that Maata Wharehoka breathes every day. It keeps her alive.

Unity

The white feather is a sign that all nations of the world will be one. Black, red, and all the others who are called human beings. This white feather is the sign of unity, prosperity, peace and goodwill.

Taare Waitara, Eulogy for Te Whiti,
November 1907

Te Whiti o Rongomai's name translates to mean the shining path of the comet. Both he and his costrategist, Tohu Kākahi, were visionaries. Te Whiti, for instance, predicted four phases or cycles in the establishment of Parihaka, all of which came to pass (Keenan 2015, 95; 195) The final phase is ongoing, as we speak. These were:

1. Takahangi or Declaration of Principles of Nonviolence. This declaration changed the course of Māori history and the history of the world. It is the birth certificate for all the nonviolent movements in the world. The declaration was completed in 1869;
2. Akarama or betrayal that occurred when agreements were violated by the Crown in 1878. Betrayal by Pākehā of commitments made to Māori are thematic. Each iteration challenges their fierce spirit of adaptation that Māori, on the other hand, never betray;
3. Tuupaapaku or Day of Grief and Loss, which was when the Parihaka community members, including Te Whiti and Tohu, were arrested and held without trial. Settlers attempted to decimate the population at Parihaka by removing and imprisoning the men who were needed for the hard work in the community, but the women rallied. Colonialists

completely underestimated their fortitude, skills, and capacity; and

4. Aranga: the resurrection, which is the truth and reconciliation process that returns to Māori what is rightfully theirs, including their language, land, resources, and dignity. This is an unfolding prophecy.

Parihaka, and the teachings of Te Whiti o Rongomai, are a provocation, an invitation, an incitement, to alchemize grief, fury, and traumatic repetition into a commitment to peace, unity, evolution, resilience, and social and environmental justice. The ways in which Te Whiti, Tohu, and everyone at Parihaka generated a relentless, unswerving cohesive focus; this is the model that Maata replicates. When you join any program at Parihaka, or attend a gathering at Te Niho, or converse with Maata, you feel the collective presence of the entire community. Your awkwardness at trying to understand a new language, your disorientation from not fully comprehending the culture, disappears as you realize that you are part of something much bigger than you and that welcomes you in. There is space for you, so you get over yourself and enjoy the grounded, loving, family spirit of Māoridom.

The legacy of tenacity and independent thinking that is in the land of Parihaka must become our collective destiny. This is where the metacrisis is pointing us; toward our innovative endurance, adaptability, and capacity to be visionary problem-solvers. The model of Te Whiti and Tohu is to never lose sight of innovative intelligence, even when the invaders are at your door. They fused traditional tikanga, or practice and belief, with what they learned and absorbed from Christianity. They evolved everything that the colonists presented to them. They brought European architecture and lighting to Parihaka. They introduced new technologies to their community. Defying any need for external validation, living by one's inner truth: that is the personal and collective model that Maata Wharehoka inherited and continues at Parihaka.

Peace

Eventually I arrived at a point in my life when I decided that being proactive was far more important to healing and building a future, and that this was inclusive of white people.

MAATA WHAREHOKA

Maata Wharehoka is a peacemaker. She helped continue the Parihaka Peace Festival, which was originally founded by Te Miringa Hohaia. The Parihaka Peace Festival was an instrument for delivering Te Whiti's messages of inclusivity and welcoming by demonstrating collaboration between Māori and Pākehā. The festivals stimulated employment possibilities for the people living at Parihaka and revealed how Māori and Pākehā could celebrate their mutuality.

The Parihaka Peace Festivals centered around artistry and innovation. They, like virtually everything that Maata creates, paraded the ingenuity that arises out of oppression. Te Whiti's strategies were creativity in action, and Tohu's articulations, the oratory that continued the oral tradition of Māori pedagogy, were also pure art. Festivals, by their nature, are unifying.

I am a Māori woman with an intense desire to heal our Māori people. I want to share the legacy of Papatūānuku, to heal our children, to heal our men who are suffering from the impacts of colonization. My

> *heart is so big. I want to help Pākehā reconcile with Māori. I want to ensure there is no blame and shame; to heal we must relinquish this behavior. I am an avid follower of Te Whiti o Rongomai. I want to see peace and harmony on all marae.*
>
> Maata Wharehoka

While all manner of horror was enacted at Parihaka, it did not destroy the possibility of the joy of a collective, a group of people acting as one. Maata's leadership is in knowing what brings people together.

Kaitiakitanga/Guardianship

Maata was mentored into her role as a guardian of Parihaka by kuia. Maata names them as her guides. "Aunty Marj Rau was my greatest role model," she says. "Through her, I built up my confidence. The woman I was, the teachings I had from my own whānau, didn't become relevant until I came to Parihaka."

In addition to Aunty Marj, Sally Karena and Ina Okeroa were mentors for Maata. "You had to work hard to live up to them," Maata acknowledges. They had high standards to uphold." These kuia trained Maata to be the kaitiaki, the caretaker, of Te Niho, one of the major community gathering and educational centers of Parihaka. By 2007, Maata and Te Ru succeeded in creating a functional, flourishing wānanga (educational center) where traditional practices were taught and where visitors were greeted with warmth and hospitality. After a long period of quiescence, Parihaka was bustling again.

The regeneration of Parihaka included the presence of the children that Maata was encouraged to bring into the world. Referring to one of her kuia aunties, Maata remembers that "Aunty Nora knew what she was doing when she asked me to have a child with Richard (Te Ru) Wharehoka." She had three!

"Soon after each birth," Maata reports, "their father took them to a nearby creek in Parihaka, in the very early hours of the morning, well before the glimmer of light could be seen on the horizon. There they were immersed and offered, in a ritual, to all the Atua and the four winds from whence they came. This iritanga was another process we revitalized and re-introduced at Parihaka."

Thus, Maata's children became part of the kaitiakitanga (guardianship) of Parihaka.

It was during this time that Maata developed her weaving skills, particularly of the mats (whāriki) that would be used for Kahu Whakatere, the burial ritual. This was no small matter. Pākehā had convinced the Māori that their traditional approach to burial was unsafe, incorrect, dangerous, and primitive. Under the influence of hegemonic domination, the Māori began to use undertakers—to turn their dead over to funeral homes. They allowed themselves to be separated from their loved ones and gave in to a dissatisfying and alienating experience of loss that left them in a state of perpetual bereavement. Maata challenged all that with Kahu Whakatere. Now, families have an alternative. Maata acknowledges, with humility: "I have helped to create a Renaissance."

Parihaka was and remains a sanctuary and a birthplace for innovation and courage. Maata articulates a commitment to make Parihaka a whakaruruhau, a haven of stability and learning, a place where families are respected and children are at the heart of everything. "I give to Parihaka my commitment to the philosophy of Te Whiti and Tohu of passive resistance and goodwill to our enemies," she declares. "This is kaitiakitanga."

For Parihaka I want to see peace and harmony in all marae. I want to know, before I die, that my work has been valued. I am an avid follower of Te Whiti o Rongomai and this leads me to promote and teach biculturalism in the home, in the workplace and in our communities. This commitment also leads me to participate actively in the preservations of Mother Earth. It is important that we rise against any further losses to what is left for Māori, and for Parihaka.

MAATA WHAREHOKA

Parihakatanga: Parihaka Consciousness

Parihakatanga is the state of consciousness that flows out of alignment with the vision put forward by Te Whiti o Rongomai of nonviolence, collaboration, inclusion, educational outreach, and peacemaking. Parihakatanga is also the commitment to delivering the message of peace globally as an Indigenous worldview. Parihakatanga is the confidence that a living, evolving wisdom stream and a redemptive, earth-centered lifestyle will bring the peace that the world longs for, in the hearts of each and every person and in the beings of all unseen dimensions.

Parihaka consciousness is imbued with love and protection for the children of Papatūānuku, the Earth Mother, and Rangi, the Sky Father. It means living in kinship with the natural world, taking a stand for sustainability, and educating people about nonviolence. Te Whiti o Rongamai was a prophet, a seer, and a brilliant strategist. He was an activist who implemented creative, nonviolent strategies with a view to the future, like the Elders, the organization founded by Nelson Mandela, for world leadership.

When Maata created the Parihaka Peace Festivals, beginning

in 2006, she did so in tribute to Te Whiti's celebratory attitude toward peacemaking. Remember that Te Whiti arranged for children to be dancing and singing, and a feast ready, when the invading soldiers arrived. This was intended to convey a message of welcome and gratitude for life that the colonizers completely ignored and misunderstood, just as Māori intelligence was disregarded. Ngapera Moeahu, principal of a Māori immersion school and resident of Parihaka, says that Maata Wharehoka *is* Parihaka. By this she means that Maata carries on the tradition that celebrates humanity through peaceful gatherings, filled with joyous creativity as the ultimate human right.

As we go through these days of the Anthropocene with splintering efforts being projected onto humanity constantly, let us remember Parihaka and the Parihaka Peace Festivals. Let us remember how the aberrations that attempted to destroy a people instead became the motivation for them to rise up and share their peacekeeping wisdom with the world.

REFLECTIONS ON PARIHAKA: REDEEMING PEACE

1. Why do you think so few people know about Parihaka? How do you understand this in the context of world history and the history of nonviolence?
2. Parihaka is a meeting ground, but it is also home to people who support and sustain it. It is a landmark, an educational resource, and where the homes and offices of individuals, like Ruakere Hond, Ph.D., a Māori scholar, are. It is also a place where regenerative agriculture and traditional cultural arts are practiced, and where a language, Te Reo Māori, is preserved, used, sustained, and evolved. Is this the kind of gathering place you would like to see in your community? Do you have such a place? Could you create it? What would it look like?
3. Parihaka is also a state of consciousness. Can you describe that consciousness?

4. How do the principles of Parihaka apply to our world today?
5. Te Whiti o Rongomai and Tohu Kākahi were true visionary leaders. Does anyone today fit that description? Describe that person and what gives them the leadership characteristics of Te Whiti or Tohu?
6. What would it take for you to become a visionary leader? Where is the community you might lead? How do you feel about envisioning yourself as a leader for that community?

3
Birthing

Ahakoa he iti, he pounamu.
Be it ever so small, it is as precious as the jade.
MĀORI PROVERB

Industrialized pregnancy and birth are highly profitable income streams for corporations and investors who capitalize on the hegemonic, culturally insensitive, authoritarian healthcare model that holds sway in the world. This model is also a primary vehicle for the colonization of minds, of life, and therefore, of the future.

In recent years, women, globally, have begun to protest the domination of their bodies, particularly in regard to pregnancy and birth. I have been part of this movement for over three decades and track it closely. I note with exuberance the increasing awareness of what Indigenous women have always embodied and the enormous value they bring to this movement. What is less well-known is that in precolonial times, women's value as the bearers of life and as wisdom keepers and leaders was highly prized.

Māori women, for instance, prioritize the understanding that their ancestors transmitted primarily through ceremony and ritual, traditionally delivered orally and practically, through daily activity, about bringing life forth. In tikanga Māori, wombs are whare tangata, the homes of the people. Tūpuna, elders and ancestors, consistently refer to the honorific passage and journeys of embryos and babies, and the mothers who carry them. Every aspect, every step, and every function of the journey to manifestation is recognized as sacred. Behind the ceremonial awareness, there is pure science. Māori birthing practices live at the precise intersection of science and spirituality. In a later chapter, I will say something quite similar about the other end of the life spectrum, or what Maata Wharehoka named *deathing.*

Of all the ways in which colonization has mined the minerals of human life, the takeover of the processes that bring life forth is the most insulting and destructive. Yet, people around the world are complicit. Looking at the etiology and duration of this confiscation, and the enormous damage it has done, I am bereft. But then, when I look up, I recognize how reclamation is now in process, and I am called to celebrate this moment in time. In particular, I celebrate Indigenous women and the resurgence of the life honoring they embody and share with us so generously.

Pregnancy, labor, delivery, and everything related to the care of children was, and remains, sacred to Māori. Women and the land are inseparable. This is exemplified in how the word for placenta is the same as the word for the land: whenua. The placenta, in fact, is not only sacred in and of itself. It is also the physiology of belonging. How the placenta is treated after birth, for instance, is of great importance to Māori, and that importance needs to be heeded by the non-Māori world. These are universal teachings. We will explore this interface in greater depth, later in this chapter. Before we do that, let's step back and look at the overall picture of what happened for women when the invasive colonizer-settlers arrived. Remember, this is Maata's back story. It is the history that shaped her and every Māori woman, as well as every Māori family.

The contrast between Māori women and settler women could not be starker. While European settlers propagated a depiction of the Māori as heathens, settler attitudes toward women and settler parental behaviors were seen as barbaric by the Māori. Māori women had greater freedom and were more respected as the bearers of children than their counterparts in Pākehā culture. And when Māori discovered that Pākehā discarded the placenta after a baby was delivered, they were horrified. This is not an antiquated past-tense contrast. It continues to this very day.

Colonizer healthcare, in order to dominate, had to name Māori practices as superstitious, even demonic. This maiming of the wisdom in Māori childbirth practices is one example of a methodical and organized manipulation of Māori minds. This systemic design to eradicate Indigenous wisdom, in healthcare and all aspects of Māori culture, is still operative. And not only in Aotearoa. Indigenous people everywhere are struggling to reclaim their wisdom streams from desecration, right now, as you read these pages.

While European women were largely identified with the private space of an indoor home, Māori women were active in all aspects of life, including trade, land ownership, farming, and as warriors. Their voices were respected in gatherings about community decision-making. At the same time, women's capacity to bring forth life and nourish the continuity of culture was prized. Māori women were regenerative practitioners, implementing and leading agricultural practices. They were military strategists. Māori women were making front-line decisions when villages were invaded by soldiers. They forged tribal alliances and were creative in navigating and circumventing the superior armaments of invasive forces. They often, if not usually, did all this while raising, feeding, and protecting children.

Today, women around the world are beginning to be recognized in these spheres, though in some countries, they still remain excluded, expelled, and restricted from them. Māori women were standard bearers of precolonial leadership, and they are starting to reclaim that status for themselves now. Maata has led the way. Everything she does restores the multifaceted mastery of Māori women. From out-front, articulate women like Maata, to the quiet kuia (elders) tending the tamariki (children), Māori women are forces of nature.

The Nest House—Whare Kōhanga

Beginning with the desire to conceive a child, there are prayers, rituals, and practices for every aspect, every step of the procreation cycle. This reflects how highly regarded pregnancy, childbearing, and child-rearing are to Māori. Barbara Brooks, writing in *A History of New Zealand Women* (2016, 35) notes how shocked Māori women were at the punitive practices that Pākehā parents used to manage their children. Māori families, in contrast, have always been affectionate and playful, and considered those who hit children *iwikino* or a bad tribe.

The whare kōhanga, or nest house, is the place built for a woman to bear her child, in the company of selected midwives, using practices passed on to the people designated for those roles. There is, in fact, a highly developed understanding of embryology, midwifery, and gynecology, including how to deliver a baby by cesarean, if necessary, in rongoā or Māori medicine. Conception, pregnancy, labor, delivery, and the immediate postpartum period are all considered to be like parts of a nest. Each phase is meant to be protected, set apart, and made holy. "Every person is sacred and requires a set of disciplines to ensure that the sacred nurturing continues," said the highly revered Rangimarie Rose Pere (1995).

Whenua/Placenta/Land

By centering Māori and other Indigenous birth wisdom in this book, I highlight their benefits to children and families everywhere, and not only for historical or anthropological value. I am speaking of benefits to the present moment. Let us look specifically at the treatment of the placenta, the afterbirth, from a Māori wisdom tradition viewpoint and contrast this with Western medical practice. I want to examine the developmental ramifications of this contrast. Consider, for instance, how adopting practices that truly understand the placenta and its role from the perspectives of science, parenting, and health, all of which are enveloped in tikanga Māori, could improve, for children and for families, what happens globally in hospital family birthing units where babies and mothers are supported by medical teams, midwives, doulas, and lactation consultants.

Hospitals typically treat placentas as medical waste or as biohazard material. From a tikanga Māori perspective, whenua (land and placenta) is not only a source of nourishment. It is also a way of knowing self, of locating self in a place and with a people. Using Western psychological terminology, the placenta is a source of formative attachment. It was, in fact, attached to us via the umbilical cord. It clearly reflects who we are, where we are, and to whom we are connected. This is why tikanga instructs parents to bury the placenta in the land. "Deposit it in the bosom of the Earth Mother, Papatūānuku" (Mead 2003, 288).

The burial of the placenta requires a ceremony. Even when separated from the child, the placenta is still part of that baby and is therefore revered. The ceremony binds the child to their homeland. Again, referencing a Western psychological model, you might say that the burial of the placenta is an act that promotes bonding. It connects the child to their roots. At the same time, the ceremony is a marker that the child has now made the transition from the darkness of the womb to *te ao mārama*, the world of light.

By all accounts, including Western science, the placenta is a miraculous organ, performing formidable functions in ways that are, to date, largely inexplicable. For instance, the placenta responds to the supply signals of both mother and child simultaneously and uses that signaling to meet the baby's developmental needs without depleting the mother. It is therefore a living biochemical conversation between mother and child within an organic structure. When Māori, and other traditional cultures, call the placenta sacred, they are referencing this microenvironment that protects all embryonic neuroendocrine systems and adapts maternal blood flow at the same time.

The placenta does all this as an independent, self-arising organ whose etiology is not completely understood. This is what is meant when the placenta is referred to as miraculous. Clearly tūpuna (ancestors) were wise physicians who knew this. It is from this pure scientific basis that they choreographed ceremonies and rituals to pay homage to the placenta, and to the relationship between baby, mother, and placenta. Contrast this with "waste" and "biohazard."

How would you feel, as a mother, if you were handed the placenta that nourished your baby in a bag marked "biohazard" and warned that it could be dangerous or infection producing? Alternately, how would you feel if you were given the gift of the placenta you cocreated with your child, in an elegant, ceremonious manner, with gratitude for its remarkable service to your family?

Maata has been speaking to these contrasts, in all aspects of healthcare for decades, including providing strategic plans for systemic change. She does this knowing the scientific basis and the developmental value of tikanga Māori. She does this as a bridge builder for all humanity, linking past and present with an eye to the future. She does this as a truth teller and seer, as a mother, grandmother, and great-grandmother, and as one who knows the power for all children in all cultures, of honoring their origins.

Esteemed Māori author Patrica Grace reports on her experience of delivering her babies in a small rural hospital in Aotearoa, in her memoir *From the Centre: A Writer's Life*. The maternity ward was run like a military base. All the mothers were in one long room, with the newborns separated in a nursery. Their screams of hunger were audible to their mothers who were not allowed to go to them. If the mothers cried for their babies, just as the babies were crying for their mothers, they were reprimanded. Placentas were incinerated without even a nod to families, sons automatically circumcised with no consent required, and the breasts of mothers bound to regulate feedings on schedule (Grace 2021, 165–166).

When Maata Wharehoka lost twins after a distressed, painful pregnancy, she was too enveloped by mourning to stop the procedures for incineration of the placenta and too vulnerable to refuse to allow the autopsies of her babies. Her father, steeped in tikanga, appeared at exactly the right moment, like a Māori Superman, to interrupt both of those procedures and retrieve the placenta, sometimes referred to as another multiple, and the twins, for honorable ceremony and burial.

Tikanga honors life. Western medicine extracts it and disposes of the evidence. If we can infuse the intention of tikanga into healthcare, we can join Maata in building bridges that benefit humanity. We can continue her lineage of courage.

By restoring the integrity and health of the placenta and the family's right to claim it as their own, Māori help us learn how to respect science and faith simultaneously. We can join them in actions like Maata's father took, actions that ultimately advocate for and protect the future of all humanity. The vicious attacks of colonization that tore tikanga Māori to shreds made deep wounds that suppurate for generations. When women like Maata and men like her father stand up in the name of life-honoring justice, they heal the pain of all Indigenous peoples.

Karanga is a welcome call, most often associated with a pōwhiri or invitation to come onto a marae. Jean Hikaka, Maata's eldest daughter, remembers how her mother taught her, before she delivered her first child, that the baby wants to hear a karanga or a karakia (prayer) of welcome from their family to greet them when they land outside the womb. Like the understanding behind the planting of the placenta in the whenua (earth), the welcoming prayer provides innate bonding and attachment, comforting and assuring a newborn, after their long, arduous journey, that they are deeply wanted by their family and their tūpuna (ancestors).

Maata also taught Jean that in advance of her baby's birth, she needed to cut a leaf of harakeke and extract the muka (fibers) to make a tie for the umbilical cord. In Te Ao Hurihuri (the ever-turning world) and Te Ao Mārama (the world of light and understanding), karanga, harakeke, and birth are always united. The muka tie is soft and gently signals the umbilicus to transition from its prenatal pulsations to life outside the womb, rather than the shock of cutting it.

Dutifully Jean did this, but when she brought the muka tie to the hospital, nurses took it away and sanitized it, not knowing that harakeke has its own antimicrobial properties. The muka was put into a small plastic bag, now no longer sacred or healing, and returned to Jean.

That was almost thirty years ago. Now, thanks to the actions of Maata and Jean, that hospital in Taranaki provides muka ties for Māori mothers-to-be and the welcoming sounds of the karanga or karakia can be heard echoing in the halls when a baby is born. This is how healthcare is reskilled by empowered women who know how to speak truth and who will settle for nothing less.

With the threads of birth and death in her hands, Maata Wharehoka weaves the whāriki (carpet) of a compassionate, respectful future civilization for all humanity.

The Children of the Future

Incorporating traditional wisdom into prenatal care, labor, delivery, birth, and postpartum care is perhaps the most effective way to prevent the atrocities of colonialism from continuing to distort this rite of passage. Reflect on the benefits for future generations of empowering babies and families to be in the center of what must be reclaimed as a miraculous life passageway. This is part of an even bigger picture of regeneration in healthcare that these times call for with great urgency.

One of the consistent values for all traditional cultures in regard to healthcare is the presence of the family. Colonized medicine designates only one authority: the physician. For Indigenous people, authority is in the collective. Many women, as a result, avoid going to physicians and to hospitals because their own reference to knowing and decision-making are automatically and instantaneously violated by strangers who obey commands that the recipients are not party to, and that may be delivered in a language they do not understand. Maata understood this so well when she advocated for changes in cervical screening for Māori women.

Babies and their families deserve to be honored. Separating a pregnant or laboring mother from her family is disrespectful. A First Nation woman in Canada described it like this: "It was hard to leave home. Leaving everyone and going on your own is harder. There's a lot of crying. Somebody should always have somebody with them to have their babies. It is hard to be alone over there to go have your babies (Neufeld and Cidro, 2017, 83)."

Women and families who have endured these insults are turning things around. For many of them, experiences like this were the impetus to reclaim traditional wisdom and pave a better way for the children of the future. Many have become active in decolonizing medicine. They are developing family birthing units grounded in traditional knowledge. They advocate for culturally safe spaces where women can reinstate collectivism and cultural rites.

Every expression of decolonization in birth is a potent declaration of possibility for the children of the future. This chapter and this book are intended to reclaim wisdom-based traditions that are rooted in pure science and adapt them for contemporary conditions. Transforming the environments for prenatal care, birth, and postpartum support, including making sure that they are culturally sensitive, transforms the future for our children.

Maata Wharehoka is devoted to children. Her poetry frequently refers to parenting and caring for children, even providing guidelines, albeit poetically. I am honored that Maata shared her poem "Who is going to take care?" with me. This poem looks to what Māori children need in order to meet the challenges of growing up in a colonized world. At the end of the poem Maata asks, "Who is going to take care when I am not there?" She beseeches parents to "step up to the mark" and not be self-indulgent because "it is the child who has to live." "Live with love," Maata implores. "Boundaries are essential but let them have a voice." That Maata uses the poetic form for this transmission is in line with the Māori tradition of oral delivery, which is, by its nature, consistently poetic, and through which teachings are remembered and recited with reverence.

In virtually all precolonial societies, motherhood was highly valued. Grandmothers, like Maata, were at the center of society.

Maata's poems and words for parents, in precolonial times, would be treated like a religious text, spiritual practice, or even a form of law. They are treasures meant to be passed on as the bylaws for the continuity of civilization. Maata resurrects and embodies this, as if recalling what her status would be in a precolonial world, and then models that remembering for other women (Nzegwu 2006, 96–97).

REFLECTIONS ON BIRTHING

1. If you go to the intersection of ceremony and science, what do you find? For instance, can you see a connection between honoring rites of passage and mental health? Please share and explore your experiences and thoughts about this.
2. What rite of passage are you ready for now? Are you birthing a new epoch in your own emergence? What is being born in you? Please commemorate it. Invite others to share this birthing with you. Choose them carefully. Document the experience.
3. Do you see a relationship between the way the medical establishment relates to birth, like incinerating the placenta, for instance, and the metacrisis environment we are in? Please describe the correlation or any thoughts and feelings you have from this reflection.
4. Western medicine has belittled and ridiculed traditional and Indigenous perspectives on birth, and on health generally. They are labeled primitive or superstitious. Can you see through this projection to a deeper understanding of practices like burying the placenta? What are the scientific and spiritual rationales for this practice, do you imagine? How do you feel about them? Do you see how they build community? What could you do, if you were motivated, to ensure these practices were included in family birthing units and culturally sensitive guidance for women?
5. Reflect on your own birth experience as a rite of passage. Do you feel it was honored as such? If not, how would you have liked yourself to be welcomed into the world?

6. Can you imagine a world in which women's wisdom about pregnancy and birth is so deeply respected that grandmothers are at the center of society and their guidance is sought with care and deep listening? Do you sense a profound value in restoring such systems and harvesting the wealth of wisdom from our elders? How can we implement this in our world today?

4
A Language of the Birds

The whole of the body speaks through the mouth.
NGĀPUHI WHAKATAUKĪ (PROVERB)

At the end, Te Puea spoke only Māori.
MICHAEL KING, *TE PUEA: A LIFE*

Puna, the first child born of the union of Maata and Te Ru, grew up at Parihaka speaking only Te Reo. Today she develops curricula to teach her language in New Zealand schools. Bubbling with life and in almost constant celebration of her language, Puna is beloved by her students. She sings and dances with them, bringing Te Reo fully alive in their blood, their bones, and in their muscles. Children of all ethnic backgrounds follow the choreographies Puna creates and that impart the messages that Te Reo has transmitted for millennia, with contemporary relevance. The veracity of that adaptation is seen in the delight her students take in their learning. Puna evolves Te Reo in the way that is innate to this remarkable, resilient language, by contextualizing every word. Like tikanga that Māori practice, Te Reo is an evolving, living being.

Maata grew up in the era when speaking Te Reo was not allowed. More than that, it was punished by beatings. Disrupting dominant culture power dynamics, Maata and Te Ru focused on fully reclaiming "their Reo." Elias and Jean were teenagers then and had to catch up. They are still bringing their Reo back into their speech and their consciousness. Today Te Reo is the language spoken on the marae. Maata's grandchildren, and the offspring of Maata and Te Ru, Puna, Te Akau, and Ngahina, were all raised speaking Te Reo as their primary language. They are fully enveloped in the cloak, the whāriki, woven from the miraculous triumph of Te Reo's survival and emergent evolution, against all the odds.

The resurrection of Te Reo reflects an intelligence that is practical and, simultaneously, thoroughly spiritual. Though originally not a written language, Te Reo was and remains poetic, lyrical, metaphoric, contextualized, and highly literary in its delivery. Rather than a literature of books, Te Reo was, and still is, a literature of song, like the language of birds.

"Te Reo is my only world, my place," Puna said to me when we met at the school where she was teaching just before the summer break in 2023. "Te Reo keeps me safe." Her sparkling, intent, dark eyes articulate her heart. She graciously shared with me her journey, beginning with her early years with Maata and Te Ru at Parihaka, a story that is a love affair with language. Later, she invited me to witness her students as they performed songs that Puna had written and dances that she choreographed to illustrate them (see figs. 4.1–4.5). Swaying, gesturing, clapping, harmonizing right alongside her students, Puna moved as one with them, clearly exhilarated. All were smiling. You could not resist it. Observers glowed with appreciation, listening intently to the performers. Their voices were vibrant, their movements so resilient they seemed to be on a trampoline. The entire performance emanated joy. It was seamless, as if it was not a performance at all but rather a way of life. This is true education.

Puna's love of Te Reo Māori is so passionate that more than

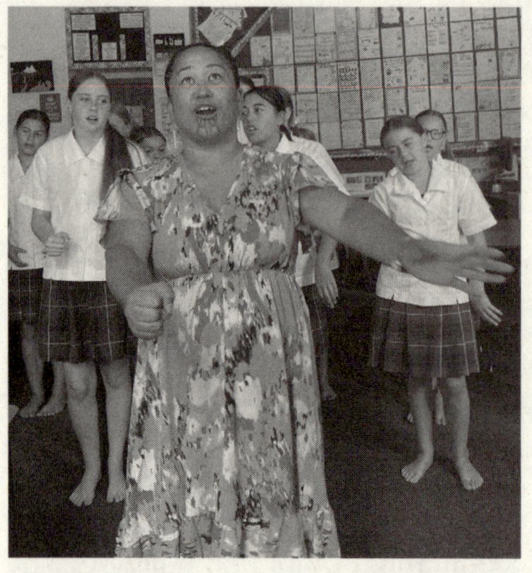

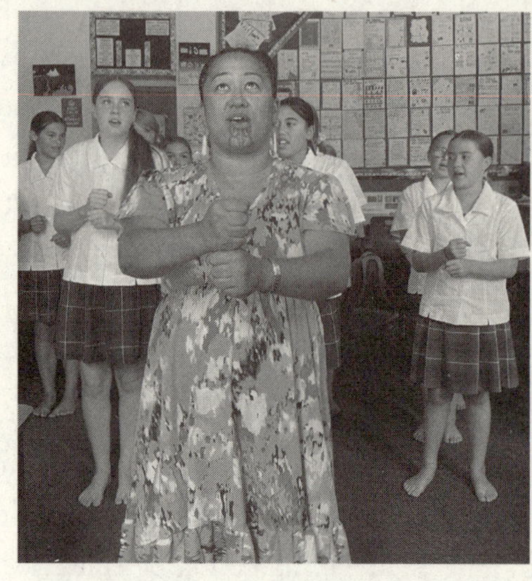

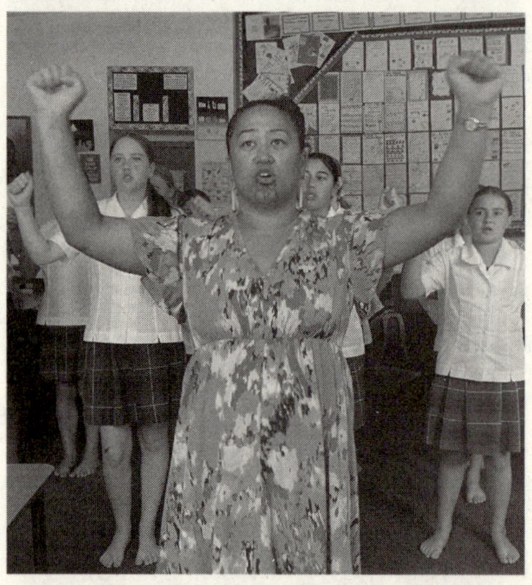

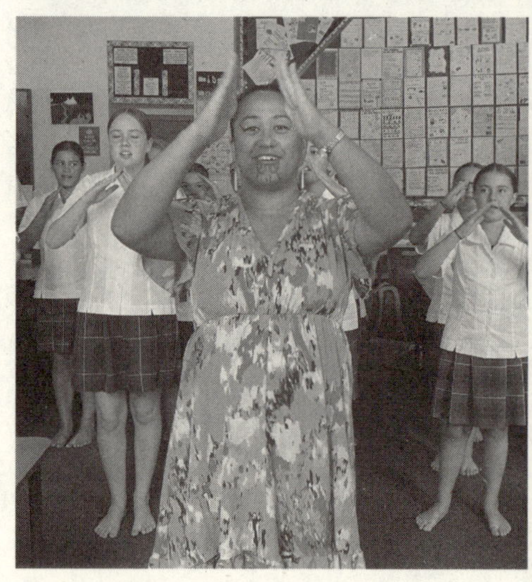

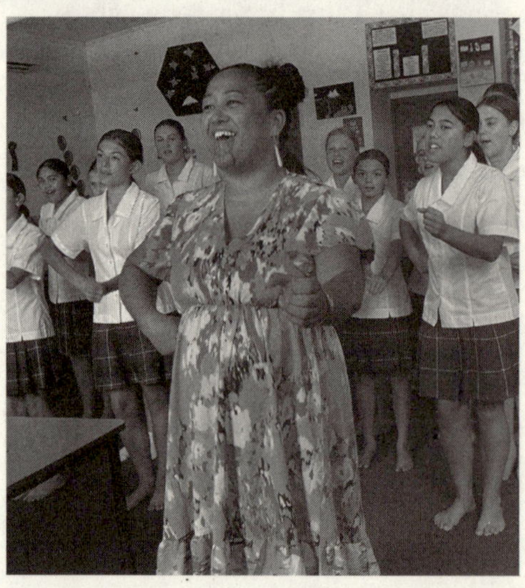

Figs. 4.1–4.5. Puna leads her class in haka

anything else, even as a teenager, she yearned to advance her knowledge and to use it in service to her people. It may be impossible for English speakers to comprehend the intimate, bonded relationship between Māori people and their language. Te Reo Māori transmits beyond the meaning of words. It carries with it Te Ao Māori, the Māori worldview. The way words are used in Te Reo conveys what it means to be Māori. The sounds soothe the body and the spirit and enliven the heart. When the settler-colonizers attempted to eradicate Te Reo, they intentionally committed an unspeakable atrocity. The wounds from this violence are still bleeding out.

Settlers saw Te Reo, just as they saw the Māori people and their practices, as primitive and unworthy of continuity. They wanted the language and the people to die and be gone, to disappear from "their" world. While missionaries, for purposes of conversion, became proficient in Te Reo, and were instrumental in converting it to a written language, they nevertheless prayed for it ultimately to be extinguished. They did not realize the impossibility of their prayers. The language and the people were as enmeshed as a mother and her newborn child or lovers who have just discovered one another.

Puna writes the songs she creates for her students, either with a pen or on a computer, whatever is handy when she is inspired and has the time and space to compose. Or she sings them into a recorder. Then these compositions are saved in a notebook, or put into a file, by her and also by others, like her students or the schools where her original compositions, her laments, hakas, dances, and refrains are presented. The performances where her compositions are given life are recorded. This documentation is new and signals a new era. Te Reo has shapeshifted from being only known through oral transmission and retained into memory, to being recorded in books, articles, recordings, videos, media, and whatever technology evolves to retain it. Te Reo takes the shape and the form needed for the current time to survive, thrive, and evolve. Te Reo Māori is a deathless being. Despite the punishing cruelty and ignorance of Pākehā, Te Reo simply could not be silenced and never will be. Each time it is spoken, Papatūānuku (mother earth) delights.

Ruakere Hond, Ph.D., a scholar of Te Reo and Te Ao Māori, and a resident of Parihaka, speaks of how Māori wisdom is recorded in waiata (songs) that entire communities learned by heart and sang together. This practice of transmitting teaching to future generations through song was not only an accepted practice. In postcolonial Aotearoa, written records were mistranslated and used to dehumanize and misrepresent Māori. In song form, however, narratives and historical recordings of events and experiences were safe (Matata-Sipu 2021, 89).

Songs sung in Te Reo, including those written by Puna Te Aroha Wharehoka, with contemporary references, are historical documents, now safe to retain in hard copies because the transcribers are Māori. This illustrates how Te Reo, the language of tangata whenua (the Māori people of the land), adapts itself to circumstances with loyalty and devotion to the intended purpose of serving the people, transmitting their beauty and heroism, their accomplishments, their challenges and triumphs, and their enduring love of their culture.

The remarkable and indomitable vibrancy of Te Reo Māori parallels the indomitable vibrancy of Maata Wharehoka. In fact, the two anneal each other. When Maata began studying Te Reo and prioritizing its use in her life and in her family, her roots grew deeper into the whenua (soil) of her new home at Parihaka. She was remaking herself. Maata had always been a strong, forward-moving, proactive woman, and now she was unequivocally all of that for Māori. The insistence on Te Reo sealed that focus. Maata's outspoken advocacy for women, for healthcare, for social, environmental, and political justice for Māori, was amplified and underscored when she became determined to do as much of that as possible in her own language, rather than in the language of the oppressor. Maata writes elegantly in English, including poetry, but the language of her spirit is Te Reo.

The explosion of women's expressive participation at all levels of global society, in what some refer to as the fourth wave of feminism, brings with it the ownership of language and voice. When Maata became Maata, discarding her previous name, Carol, she modeled for other women the transformative potential of clearly proclaiming selfhood and agency. The women around her took note.

Maata's granddaughter, Hotukura Wharehoka, wrote her doctoral thesis on ingoa tangata, or Māori names, and how their reclamation is a demonstration of self-determination. It was Maata who resurrected traditional naming practices, just as she resurrected traditional birthing and deathing practices. Maata transmitted that wisdom to Hotukura, who has consummated her learning not only in her published doctoral thesis (Seed-Pihama 2017) but in her family and community life. As a professor, she is a vociferous advocate for ingoa tangata and Te Reo Māori. She is infused with Maata's legacy.

Hotukura asserts in her thesis that the reclamation of traditional language and naming practices is integral to well-being. Healing happens when you oppose the hegemonic forces by which colonizers confiscate language or make Indigenous words and names unimportant. Pākehā attempted to erase personal names for Māori, along with their names for plants, mountains, rivers, places, and everything that had been consecrated by Māori naming rituals like structures, homes, and rooms.

Can you see the broad ramifications of reclaiming one's name? As the descendant of immigrants, I can testify to the long-term impacts of my name being mispronounced and ultimately changed to another name so that English speakers could say it without effort; without making them uncomfortable. A woman told me recently about how a chronic illness that plagued her as a child ended, virtually instantaneously, when her dying grandmother who immigrated from the Middle East insisted that her surviving granddaughter revert to her given name rather than the name imposed on her by others from the dominant culture.

Kuiatanga: Elder Women as Vessels of Language Fluency and Self-Determination

Binding me to my culture is my language.

MAATA WHAREHOKA

While women won the right to vote in 1893 in New Zealand, they could not stand for Parliament until 1919, and it was not until 1949 that a Māori woman, Iriaka Ratana, became a member of Parliament. Nevertheless, long before that, women played a central role in movements to integrate Māori into New Zealand governance and to reclaim Māori land rights. For this to be so, Māori women had to become bilingual. Fluency and outspoken advocacy came quickly and easily for Māori women, but it necessitated adaptation. Powerful Māori women were anathema to colonialists. Suppression of their language and cultural practices, like the traditional moko kauwae (chin and lip tattoos) was required in order for Māori women to be successful advocates for their people. Thanks to women like Maata, who proudly wears her moko kauwae, this identity practice is being restored.

In 1892, the Māori formed their own Parliament, Te Kotahitanga, and from the inception, women were active and outspoken. Though they could not stand as members, Māori women could speak in their Parliament, in contrast to the New Zealand Parliament where Pākehā women could not speak.

The women formed Ngā Komiti Wahine, a national network of tribally based Māori women's committees. They addressed domestic violence, treatment of solo mothers, smoking, alcohol consumption, retention of traditional Māori women's skills, and religion. They spoke freely about these issues in their own language, and then shared beyond their groups in English. Niniwa I te Rangi of Wairarapa, a member of Ngā Komiti Wahine, started a bilingual newspaper, produced and fully staffed by Māori women. Finally, in 1897, women won the right to vote and stand for the Māori Parliament. Te Reo Māori has now found its way into Parliament. I predict that one day in the not-too-distant future, there will be a Māori Wahine (Woman) Prime Minister.

Even when feeling unwell, Maata Wharehoka's voice rings out with the chants that call the family to a meal or when visitors are welcomed. Like the reclamation and re-emergence of Kahu Whakatere (rites for death and dying) portrayed in the deathing chapter of this book, and ingoa tangata (naming practices), the reclamation of language is an epic, even mythic, statement about sovereignty. These cultural ways of being, embedded in the Māori language, are the birthright of every Māori person and are carried in the bodies of the kuia, the women elders, like Maata, and delivered through them to their whānau (families), iwi (tribes), and hapū (communities or subtribes). Even when forced to suppress Te Reo, it was retained in the flesh of the kuia for safekeeping, along with every cultural treasure of the Māori people. This is one of the primary reasons that kuia (elder women) are revered in Māori communities.

Women throughout the world, and especially elders, would do well to be inspired by this and recall their innate lineage-holding capacity through the eggs that are passed from one grandmother's generation to the next. If women could universally translate this knowing into voicing truth, it could change the world. I predict that it will.

The British deliberately targeted women in their colonial onslaughts because they knew that this was the fastest route to damaging Māori social organization. Rape was a strategy beginning with Captain Cook's crew and in the vicious attack on Parihaka. (See the chapter in this book devoted to Parihaka.) Prior to colonization, Māori women were landholders, warriors, navigators, and political and spiritual leaders. Given the specific targeting to humiliate and disempower them, it is worthy of note that tenacious women like Maata Wharehoka use their language to restore dignity and leadership to wahine Māori (Māori women). This is what is meant by kuiatanga.

Colonizers did not see women, even Pākehā women, as valid knowledge holders. White ethnographers and historians perpetuated that ignorance by not speaking of them. To this day, the common assumption is that knowledge belongs to men. Yet within Māori life, women are known as the true keepers of wisdom. The kuia, elder women, are the protectors, the ones who sustain and impart lineage stories. They embody the history and origin of names within a family and even a community, and particularly on the marae. They are the ones who tell the birthing stories that gave rise to those names. The true narratives, untold for too long, that kuia and elder women everywhere know, are needed to reclaim the power of humanity. Indeed, the world longs to hear them.

Language, Names, Birth, and Identity

> *I've learned my name. I rise. I rose up. I remembered it. Now I could tell my story. It was different from the stories told about me.*
>
> Eavan Boland

When she met and married Te Ru Koriri Wharehoka, Maata found a partner in her dedication to the future of the Māori. Nowhere was this more evident than in their parenting. Maata speaks about how Te Ru responded to the births of his children.

> *Soon after their birth, their father took them to a creek, in the very early hours of the morning, well before the glimmer of light could be seen on the horizon, where they were immersed and offered, in a ritual, to all the Atua and the four winds from whence they came. The iritanga, a process revitalized, now practiced in Taranaki.*
>
> MAATA WHAREHOKA

Maata Wharehoka has taken a stand for her people by advocating for them to enter the world knowing they are Māori, and exit the world knowing they are Māori. She also takes a firm stand that whānau (family) be directly engaged at these critical times so that the baby and the person transitioning from life know not only who they are but who is there to support and nourish them. That these rites of passage be conducted in Teo Reo, and that the names of the newly born or newly departed be reiterated in Te Reo, is essential for those living, those in the other dimensions, for the tamariki (the children), and for Papatūānuku (mother earth).

Maata formed her understanding of these practices from studying tikanga (traditional Māori practices), yet these fundamental concepts of birthright, identity, language, and community apply to everyone. When Maata Wharehoka brings them into consciousness for Māori, the entire world benefits.

Whenua

The whenua is the medium between the mother and child, succoring a new life. After birth, the whenua, as land, succors the whānau.

Hirini Moko Mead, *Tikanga Māori*

Te whare tangata is both in the womb of our mothers and mirrored in another house of humankind—the new world of light into which we are born.

Hotukura Wharehoka

The identity imparted through Māori naming and Te Reo Māori is summed up in the word whenua (placenta, land) and in the designation of Māori as tangata whenua (the people of the land). Everything comes together when we see that tangata whenua also refers to the place where the umbilical cord is buried, and that the other major meaning of the word *whenua* is the womb. Please read more about this in the chapter on birthing in this book.

Everything in Te Ao Māori is about belonging. Language inscribes that belonging into the fibers of our being. Names, including place names, plant names, and the names given to children born into a world where they can be first-language speakers of Te Reo, all create a caul of protection for the legacy of Te Ao Māori. Parenting for belonging is Maata's model for how to grow up Māori in this world, asserting and re-asserting the dignity of being Māori, claiming it and reclaiming it in every action and with every word.

Speaking Te Reo is like stepping into a verdant landscape in which humans and plants, animals, the land, the wind, the rain, the mountains, and the rivers are all united, blended, operating from the same intentionality. This is the model of connected living that

Maata Wharehoka, and others like her, deliver, and they do this for everyone, as well as for their children and their grandchildren. They do this for all the children of the future. Their model inspires us to stand up for who we really are and speak the language of our souls.

REFLECTIONS ON LANGUAGE AND CULTURE

1. In reading about Puna's love affair with her language, do you feel any resonance with your own language? How much of your identity is transmitted through your use of your language? Please explore and share your experience of identity and language.
2. What do you know about the origins of your name? Tell the story of your name and how you received it.
3. Some people change their names. Have you ever considered this? What name really reflects who you are and how you experience yourself in the world?
4. Are you multilingual? Do you have an experience of one language that expresses your essential self? Share about these experiences of language and selfhood.
5. Do you notice that you feel and move differently when you speak different languages? Explore this. What does it tell you about the physiology of language?
6. What is the language of your lineage? Is that the language you speak? Do you speak a language that was imposed on you? Describe what it is like to speak a language because you have to, and if you never had such an experience, imagine what that would be like for you and describe that.
7. Have your thoughts, understandings, perceptions about language and names changed as a result of reading this chapter? How?

5

Toi Māori: Informed by Spirit

Māori art originates in the celestial realm.

Julie Paama-Pengelly

Maata Wharehoka is a multifaceted artist. She writes poetry, paints, and weaves, to name just a few of the forms she employs. As her son Te Akau says, she can master any art form she chooses. She is a self-taught artist, and the recipient of the Te Waka Toi Award from Creative New Zealand. This book shares Maata's artistry with the world.

Maata is also a healing artist and a creative community organizer and speaker. The impetus behind all of her expressions is her self-declared passion for her people. Māori art always conveys knowledge and values. It is pure pedagogy.

Māori traditions were not recorded in writing. This is an essential awareness in understanding Māori art and specifically in understanding Maata Wharehoka's consuming drive to create and to share her creativity. She is motivated by the mantle she describes herself as carrying. That mantle is constructed by Te Ao Mārama, the world of knowledge and light.

"The origin of original art forms is attributed to ancestors who overcame certain obstacles in order to acquire art knowledge from the deities, or atua, so that the requisite skills and information could be made available to those in the mortal world," says Julie Paama-Pengelly in her book *Maori Art and Design* (2010). Maata instinctively embodies this tradition. Everything she creates, she says, is "informed by spirit."

The esteemed Rangimarie Rose Pere, who died in 2020, said to Maata when she visited Parihaka, "Maata, I want you to heal Papatūānuku." In everything that Maata creates, this directive echoes as the intention and purpose of her artistry in all its many forms.

Māori art is simultaneously breathtakingly beautiful and eminently practical. This is exemplified in the creation and manifestation of Kahu Whakatere, which is, each time it is experienced, living art. "When we need something, we create it," Maata said. "And we needed Kahu Whakatere." It is a nexus of creative and cultural expressions. It is also Maata's consummate, quintessential artistic creation. Therefore, it is referenced in this book in several sections. An entire chapter is devoted to its role as tikanga, or cultural practice. Here I would like to explore it as toi Māori, as a Māori artform.

Kahu Whakatere

In the invalidation and desecration of Māori practices and language, colonization actively and intentionally smothered the very souls of Māori people, suffocating their voices and misrepresenting Māori traditions. In silencing Māori ritual, expression, language, rites of passage, art, and education, a violent and abusive theft was committed. All of Maata's art and her advocacy for Te Reo (Māori language), Māori education, healthcare, and social services, is to reclaim the dignity and beauty of her people. That she does this with such unwavering and persistent self-confidence is her hallmark. Nowhere is this more evident than in the manifestation of Kahu Whakatere. This contribution reverberates in meaning and value for the entire world.

When Maata brought her eldest sister home to Parihaka because she was dying, she was confronted with the fact that Māori death and dying rituals had become virtually extinct. They had been replaced completely by Pākehā (European) practices of funerals, embalming, and burial.

Maata and her husband Te Ru determined not to follow these Pākehā practices, but to reinstate, reinvigorate, and even innovate, the Māori way. Because Māori practices were never documented in writing, details had been lost through the silencing and other punitive and degrading forces of colonization. Maata and Te Ru would not accept this erasure of their history, so they reinstated and reinvented traditional practices. With this uppermost in their minds and attuning to what they felt was right for Maata's sister, Maata and Te Ru creatively and collaboratively rebirthed the practices for death and dying for her, and then realized they were doing that for themselves, for their family, for their community, and for all Māori. I suggest that Maata and Te Ru were doing this for all humanity. The entire world needs to understand loss, grief, death, and dying, in a way that is informed by Indigenous wisdom. That is the contribution of Kahu Whakatere that makes death and dying into a work of great art. Kahu Whakatere is the epitome of toi Māori.

When Te Ru Wharehoka became severely ill and was dying, he gave his passage, his transition, to the further evolution of what he and his wife had begun. Maata completed the design for and with her husband, alongside their children, during his end days and after his passing. Kahu Whakatere has now served hundreds of families in Aotearoa New Zealand. It is being maintained and sustained by

Maata's children with her guidance now, and they will continue her transmission after her passing.

Kahu Whakatere is a ritual process for what Maata calls *deathing*. She invented that word to equate it with *birthing*. Kahu Whakatere is a comprehensive work of art, and Maata has overseen every aspect of it. The weaving of the mats and the garments is envisioned, designed, and created by her. Specific waiata (songs), chants, and prayers (karakia) are orchestrated to honor the departed loved one who leaves the earth plane surrounded by love, community, and culture.

Kahu Whakatere implements the Māori world view. It is informed by beauty, respect, and love. It is of service to the people. It conveys wisdom teachings. The entire process is values informed, beginning with the prayers that set the intentions of the ceremony, and the harvesting of the harakeke (flax) for weaving. Kahu Whakatere is living pedagogy, transmitting wisdom, traditions, and beliefs to younger generations who are always involved, even if they are simply playing nearby. Bobbing in and out, entering the room for contact, for food, to watch, or to share something, the little ones absorb the intentions of the ritual. Everything is for them, and everything is for the community. This is the nature of all Māori art.

The harakeke weavings in various forms serve a multiplicity of purposes, not the least of which is to surround the grieving family with beauty and to engage them in healing practices. As whānau (family members) weave, they impart their memories, their celebrations, their emotions, their laughter, their hopes, and shared dreams, their personal, most intimate experiences with the departed loved one, into the mats upon which that person will lie and into the garments that person will wear in the rite of passage for the soul and spirit of their being.

The silky threads of the harakeke are the tassels, the curtains, the filaments through which the soul departs on a journey woven by those with whom they shared life. One person who spoke of the Kahu Whakatere process for her brother told me how she lay beside his body, dressed in a garment woven by his siblings, just as she had laid beside him as a very small child. She remembered their nights of laughter and playfulness, and all the moments of childish delight that they had shared. She bid farewell to his body swathed in the treasures of their relationship, a smile upon her face just as genuine as her tears. This is art of the highest order.

Every component of Kahu Whakatere is of the land where the departed experienced life. The land, the whenua, is where they return. The people who touch them, clean, prepare, and clothe them for their final journey back to the whenua, are the people who shared the foundational moments of their existence, not strangers. Every touch is familiar. No chemicals, no embalming, no clinical environment to startle the soul and the spirit.

Kahu Whakatere embraces one person's life and one person's death, but it also honors the entire family of the departed, giving them acts of beauty, transformation, and comfort to perform. This eases and fully integrates the loss of their loved one, without ever abandoning that being whose life has now been fulfilled.

With each Kahu Whakatere that is enacted, the soul of the Māori people, ravaged and eviscerated by colonialism, is restored to its original dignity and connection with Papatūānuku, our mother earth. In this way, what Maata has created honors the directive she received from Rangimarie Rose Pere.

In every Kahu Whakatere, the departed one is held and acknowledged as tangata whenua (person born of the land). Each being is precious to the people, like babies are precious, as birth is precious. The preciousness of death is restored through the burial ritual and the way of the people is resurrected. Every strand of the mats and garments of Kahu Whakatere is woven with this peace.

The resurgent beauty of Māori art, the sweet storytelling within the weaving, is a triumph over violence and loss. That this art continues and evolves, just as Maata Wharehoka generates new weaving designs, and new ways of weaving, just as she writes poetry and paints, is a tribute to the unifying and regenerative, enduring, and triumphant power of Māori art, of toi Māori.

Toi Māori, Māori art, is always considered to be collaborative. Even if only one person makes the art, there is a collaboration with tūpuna (ancestors). Often a work of art is the product of many hands, and when it is, there is no insistence on crediting anyone in particular. Artists give their creativity willingly and generously to toi Māori.

I watched Maata insist once, as a group of weavers gathered around her to help complete a project, that each one of them sign their names on their weaving contribution, even if it was just a small mat, or a portion of a larger weaving. She wanted everyone to know that this project was a collective effort, from and for the community, and not hers alone, though she knew she would receive the attention and the credit. These weavers had come from all over Aotearoa because Maata needed their help. Many were expert weavers, and others came to learn from them. They had dropped everything to weave for and with Maata because they love and revere her. Each one felt that it was an honor to be asked by Maata Wharehoka to join in a project that she initiated.

While Kahu Whakatere sums up the meaning of Māori art, and what all of the artistry of Maata Wharehoka intends, it is simultaneously a teaching for the world. As the old story of extraction, colonialism, domination, and racism dies, a possibility of unity, peace, and love is woven by Kahu Whakatere. We inhabit a time of dramatic death and rebirth. The art of Maata Wharehoka, while it reaches into the traditions of her culture, also extends itself forward, to a future that will unfold past her life, into the lives of her children, her grandchildren and her great-grandchildren, and all Māori children. Maata's vision extends into a world where Māori art will thrive and be received by more and more people, beyond Aotearoa. There is no doubt that Maata Wharehoka is a seer, a visionary. The peace and unity that she sees is in every work of art she makes, inspires, intends, and delivers. Her greatest work of art, let it be said here and now, is her life.

Mum can make something out of nothing.
NGAHINA AND TE AKAU WHAREHOKA

Te Akau, Maata's youngest son, attributes Maata's visionary capacity to her early upbringing in rural Tauranga, in a poor family. "She had to be resourceful," he says. "And this unlocked her creativity. She had to picture things in order to create them and make them happen. And now she is a kuia (elder), and she can be creative at the drop of a hat."

"Mum comes from a generation with a high and tough standard," Te Akau continues. We are sitting outside the wharenui where he and his family live with Maata, on a hot summer day. We have been weaving together for an exhibit of Maata's designs for Kahu Whakatere. Maata's high standards of accomplishment and performance," Te Akau says, "is dying." Nevertheless, Te Akau and his siblings understand what the leadership that Maata passes to them requires. They are committed to sustaining those standards. "We have grown up with it," he says. "We have seen how to balance the world of old with what is happening now. We will never let go of what Mum has taught us, and we can evolve it, just as she has evolved traditional teachings."

"There is a stubbornness," both Te Akau and his sister Ngahina say, to Maata's lifestyle. "She doesn't ask for help. She figures how to do everything herself." The new generation of Wharehoka leadership is adapting to another, more contemporary, era, but without losing sight of the past. Ngahina is also extremely creative, and she sometimes challenges tradition. "We come from a different outlook. We have been raised in the revitalized Māori world. We have a bond to our language and our land that is given to us at birth, unlike my mother, who had to fight hard to revitalize that connection."

"The most honorable thing we can do for Māmā and Pāpā is to live this Māori life in our way," Ngahina says. "They gave us adaptability, and we will sustain our lineage confidently, in our own way."

"My mum is the voice of our ancestors," Te Akau says. "And she is unwavering in that. I have grown up with that wisdom and that model. Everything we do has a genealogy. We have the fortune to have lived with that, and we see what our ancestors saw, through my mother's life and her art. We are fortunate that our mother held onto that. It is the little things, such as the way you serve a meal or make a bed for your visitors. It is in everything that we do. Art is life."

Toi Māori

> *In traditional Māori belief a talent for creativity comes to the individual through one's ancestry.*
>
> Hirini Moko Mead

Maata's art is Maata's heart. It is her restoration. It is her expression. It is deeply personal. Through her poems and her visual art, it is possible for those who have not met Maata Wharehoka, who have not been in her physical presence, to feel the raw power of this woman who is a force of nature. Maata is a woman who has built a bridge from the past to the future with her art. This bridge is not only for Māori to walk. It is for all of us because we have all been colonized, and we all need her model of reclaiming the truth of who we are. Maata is a woman who loves all children, a mother, a grandmother, and a great-grandmother whose undiluted love for her people is her legacy. This proverb is as if written specifically for her:

Kia whakatōmuri te haere whakamua.
I walk backward into the future with my eyes
fixed on the past.

Maata's self-portrait (see plate 3) and her portrait of her husband (see plate 4), Te Ru Wharehoka, known fondly to many as Pāpā, speak volumes about their strength, their intensity, and their unfailing commitment. Remember that Maata is a self-taught artist. She delivers Pāpā, who was a tōtara, a great one, to the world through her portrait of him. She shares her sense of self through her self-portrait. Her portrait of Maunga Taranaki (see plate 5), the other man in her life, comes from how she views him in her soul.

It is through her poetry that Maata allows herself to grieve. A tower of light, Maata carries in her body the keening of her magnificent people. Maata Wharehoka is the container of all that it means to be kuia, to be a Māori wahine, to be an elder who knows in her blood and in her bones the secrets of her people, their undying courage and their faith.

This poem, which Maata leaves untitled, but which I would call a lament, speaks volumes of what courses through the sinews of Maata

Wharehoka's being every moment of her life. The poem, as I perceive it, is like a song, a wailing outcry that we must not turn from, that we must heed.

Stolen, stolen
My land
My land stolen
My land stolen, taken
Stolen, lost to the white man
Stolen
My land stolen.

It will be forgotten
No one wants to remember
But live on my children
Into a world of greed and theft
No one wants to know
How much it hurts
Especially those who have stolen.

It is not a forgotten story
Live with this in your hearts
Make it live in your mokopuna
Forever forever.

Never let it be forgotten
Else the world we live in
Will be nothing.
Live to be Māori
Forever and ever
Don't live with the hate

Our parents lived with
But keep alive the
Land that was stolen.

There lies your history
Your history
For the world to know
The white man came with intent to take
With intent to gain
With intent to destroy
With intent to be the power
The power that should be you.
Whina "we are one"
Hone "get a life live in the 20th century"
Te Ru "hold on to what is Māori"
The people "the only thing Māori
Is our powhiri"
"Even our own people
Want the god damn thing in English"
Learn well
Shakespeare "out, out damn spot"

I like that.
Know the world
It fits into your palm
Carry it with you wherever you go
Change what needs to be changed
But don't change the Māori.
Get back what has been stolen.

MAATA WHAREHOKA

I heard Maata comment to her friends one evening in her kitchen, as we sat around her abundant table after a day of weaving, that she was hearing voices from the other side of this dimension, calling to her. The other women nodded with understanding, everyone acknowledging wordlessly that we were sharing the last days or weeks, maybe months or perhaps years of Maata's life.

We felt the breath of the spirits who were whispering to Maata. We heard them murmuring in our ears, and each one of us treasured our auspicious moments with her. We clung to her. She was so alive and close to us now. We wanted her to continue leading us, to continue modeling what it meant to be a strong Māori woman.

We wanted Maata to show us how to be in the end days, just as she had shown us the way in life. We knew we could rely on her to tell us the straight up truth of what would come for all of us, just as she always told us the straight up truth about life. In her pain and with the fragility of the tenuous nature of her life as she struggled to breathe and walk, Maata still inspired us, as she always had. We knew that until her last breath, and probably long after, she would challenge us with her fantastic, demanding, and feisty love. We never wanted that to end.

Maata's poem "Karanga" speaks to this attunement she has to what is beyond this plane, the way in which she is informed by spirit, and has been from the moment she entered the world.

Oh my God!
Not really!
But oh yes, it is so

That call Māori women give
A reminder of the old people
Makes the blood curdle sometimes

Especially when there is a call from the belly of bellies
And the endless song of waiting for the visitor.

The visitor slips in and out resting here and there
Gently stroking the brow
There's a gentle wafting of a fragrance
Familiar to me when my Aunt passed on
White flowers, thousands of them
She leaves without bidding me farewell.

No, I am not too sure I stay around to see or hear again
But I do and I breathe silently while I wait in anticipation
I know I long for the guidance of any of them
They karanga just like my Aunty did
No not like that; not that screaming high-pitched sound
Just a gentle cooeeeeeeee
Coooooooooeeeeeee

Now that's the hair thriller
Not being prepared
Waiting for the moment
The right moment
Then they are gone
Speed
Lightning speed
Gone
Gone for ever.

MAATA WHAREHOKA

Maata's dedication to children, to Te Ao Māori informed parenting, to honoring tikanga in the interest of children's well-being, infuses her poetry, as if all of it was written as encouragement and guidance for adults to steward the little ones. Her poem "Lying and Cheating and Stealing" speaks to that. You can hear Maata's cautionary, instructive voice clearly in these stanzas, along with her community-minded faith that together we can make the world a better place.

Believe me I wouldn't have made my mind up
this way
If you told me the truth from the beginning,
Cos kiddo lying and cheating and stealing
I never did like.

You need to know that there are too many
people
Cheating their way through life.
They make the best criminals
And they destroy families.

Their values and beliefs do not fit.
They make the world a sad place for kids
Who don't need to be led by cheaters and
stealers.
They need the kind of lead that helps them
Grow into citizens who can make the next
person happy.

So don't ever leave the child minded by the
evil.

Make it a great world for all of us.
Hand them a hand that is full of care.
Walk with them so they cannot fall.

Show them the way that is made for eternity.
Give them the words so they may utter
goodness.
Teach them so that they live in wellness.
Stand by them whenever they fall.

MAATA WHAREHOKA

There seems no better way to honor a poet of the caliber of Maata Wharehoka than by offering her a poem, which I would like to do here.

*Kaitiakitanga**

FOR MAATA WHAREHOKA

Women weave the world into being.

SHARON BLACKIE

Dedicated to the unity of all women.
My fierce, rooted Māori Sister,
You defy the theft of your land.
You exhale the breath of life into the world.
You fill your people with staunch, enduring love.
I carry your transmission
In the basket you have woven,
The basket of fibrous soul.

STEPHANIE MINES

---

*Kaitiakitanga: Stewardship

REFLECTIONS ON MAATA'S MODEL
For Artists and Creatives

1. If your art was intended to serve your community as well as your own personal expression, how would it change?
2. How is your artistic expression reflective of a collective experience as well as your personal experience?
3. When you consider your audience, who do you see? Do you see a diverse population, or people who look like you?
4. Does your choice of expressive, artistic mediums have a lineage from your culture or your family? If so, how do you acknowledge that in your creativity? If this is not the case, why is that?
5. How do the materials you use in your creative expression suggest a relationship to your culture?
6. Think of your creativity and expression in regard to your legacy. When you do that, does it change your expression, or shift it in some nuanced way? Explain please.
7. How natural is your voice in your creative expression? Maata Wharehoka models being purely herself in all her art, whether it be visual art, poetry, or community organizing. This takes great daring and confidence. Have you found that capacity within yourself? Would you like to embody it? How can you secure this genuine, authentic voice and use it?

6

He Wahine He Taonga: Every Woman Is a Treasure

There's a glass ceiling for women generally, and then there's a lower, in-house ceiling that's actually for Māori women.

LEONIE PIHAMA

Women's empowerment is never as simple as personal choice, because people face multiple layers of discrimination that interact to make the world a harder place in which to move forward.

MICHELLE DUFF

Maata Wharehoka's pioneering efforts in healthcare, parenting, and social and racial justice were ahead of her time. She was already speaking and acting as the fourth wave of feminism that acknowledges intersectionality when she was a teenager. Her lineage will be carried into the future by those who read this book, by her family, and by the thousands of Māori women she has influenced. Perhaps when New Zealand has a Māori wahine (woman) prime minister, we will realize even more widely the fruits of her mahi (efforts).

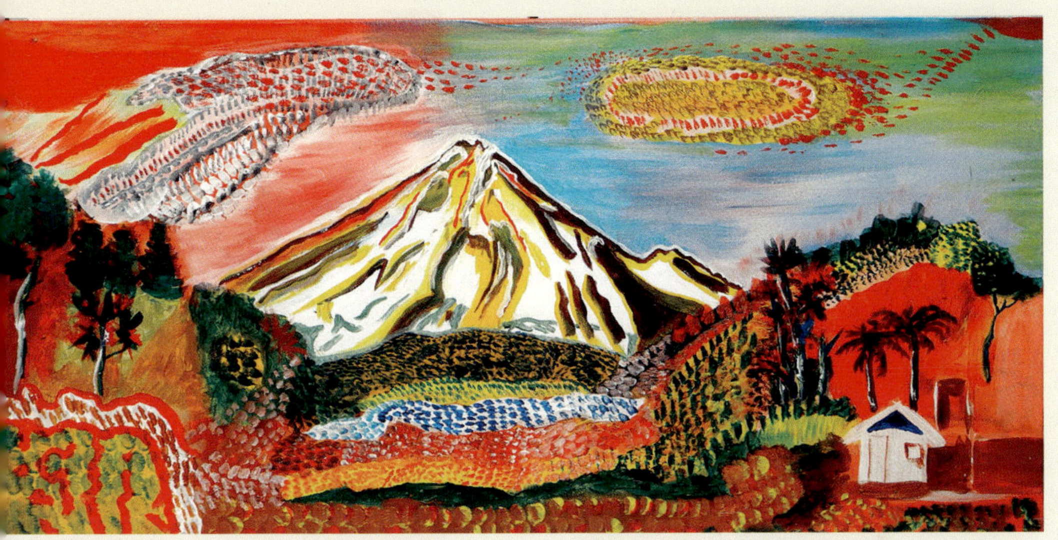

Plate 1. Maunga Taranaki with Parihaka in the foreground
Painting by Maata Wharehoka

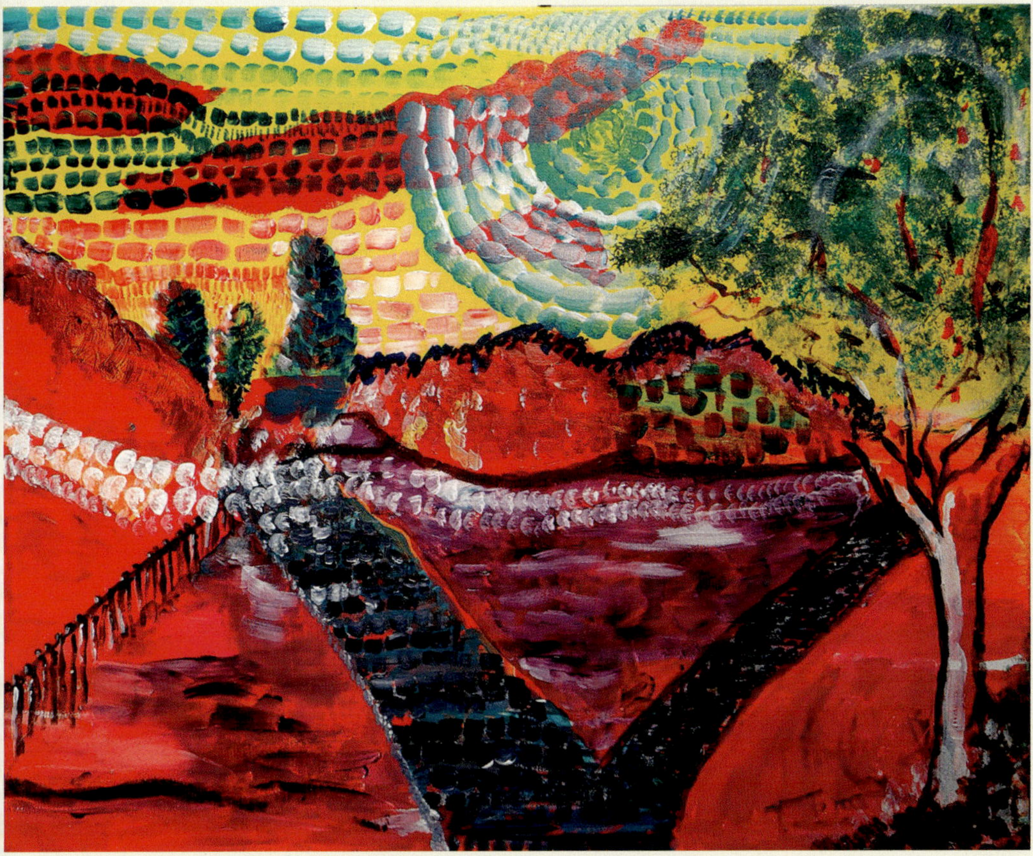

Plate 2. Entrance to Parihaka
Painting by Maata Wharehoka

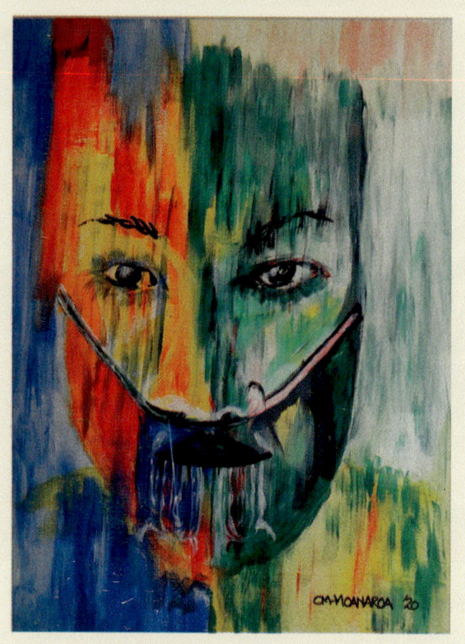

Plate 3. Self-portrait
Painting by Maata Wharehoka

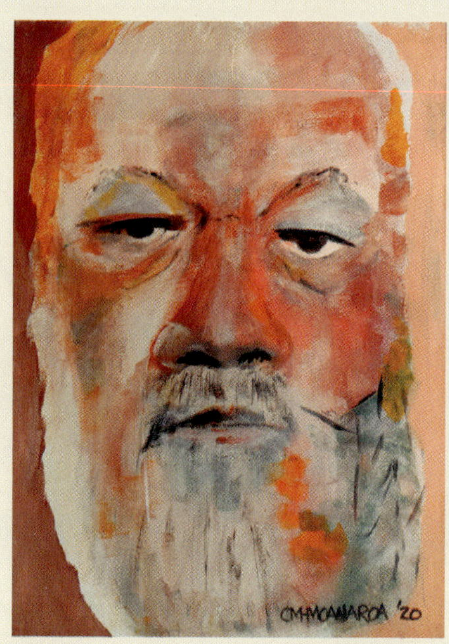

Plate 4. Portrait of Te Ru Wharehoka
Painting by Maata Wharehoka

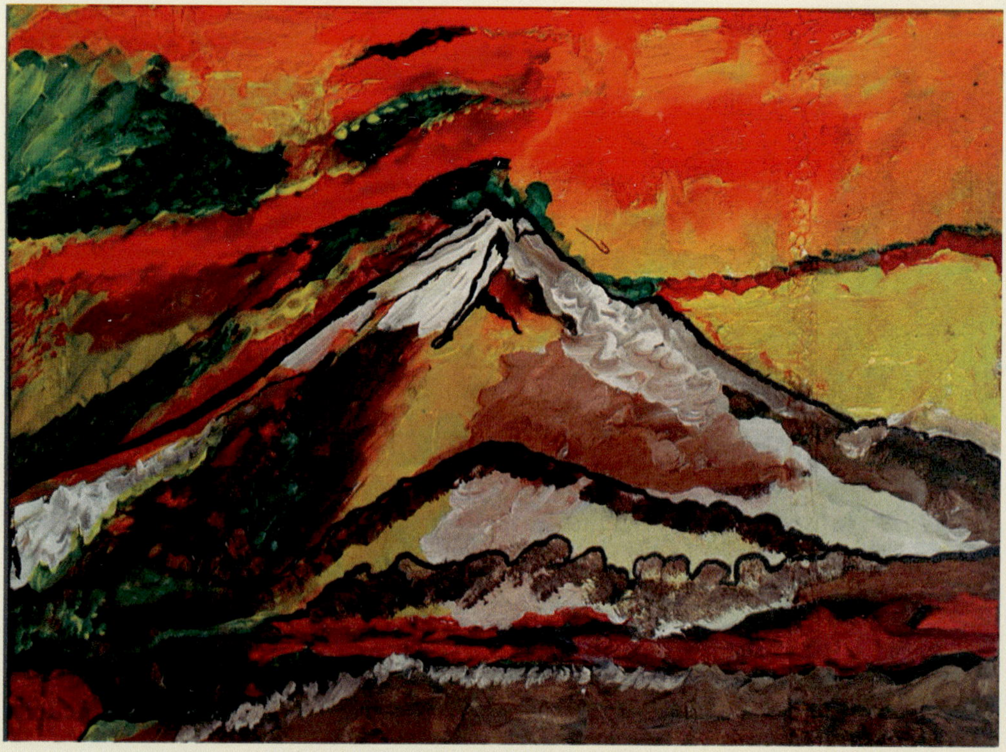

Plate 5. Maunga Taranaki
Painting by Maata Wharehoka

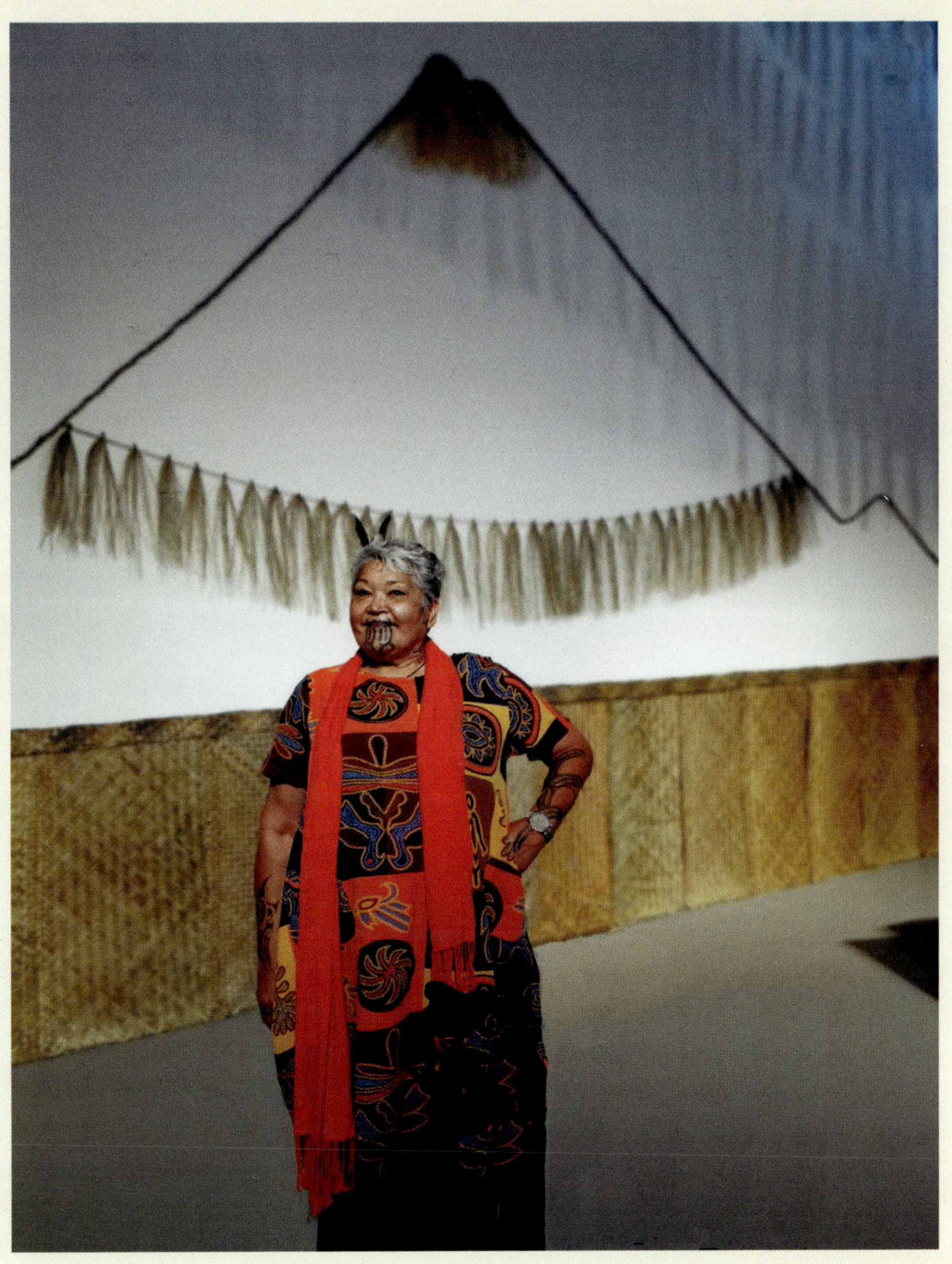

Plate 6. Maata Wharehoka stands in front of *Fibrous Soul*
Photo by Jean Hikaka

STOP!
ALL VISITORS MUST READ
THIS NOTICE
PARIHAKA
COVID19
MARCH 2020

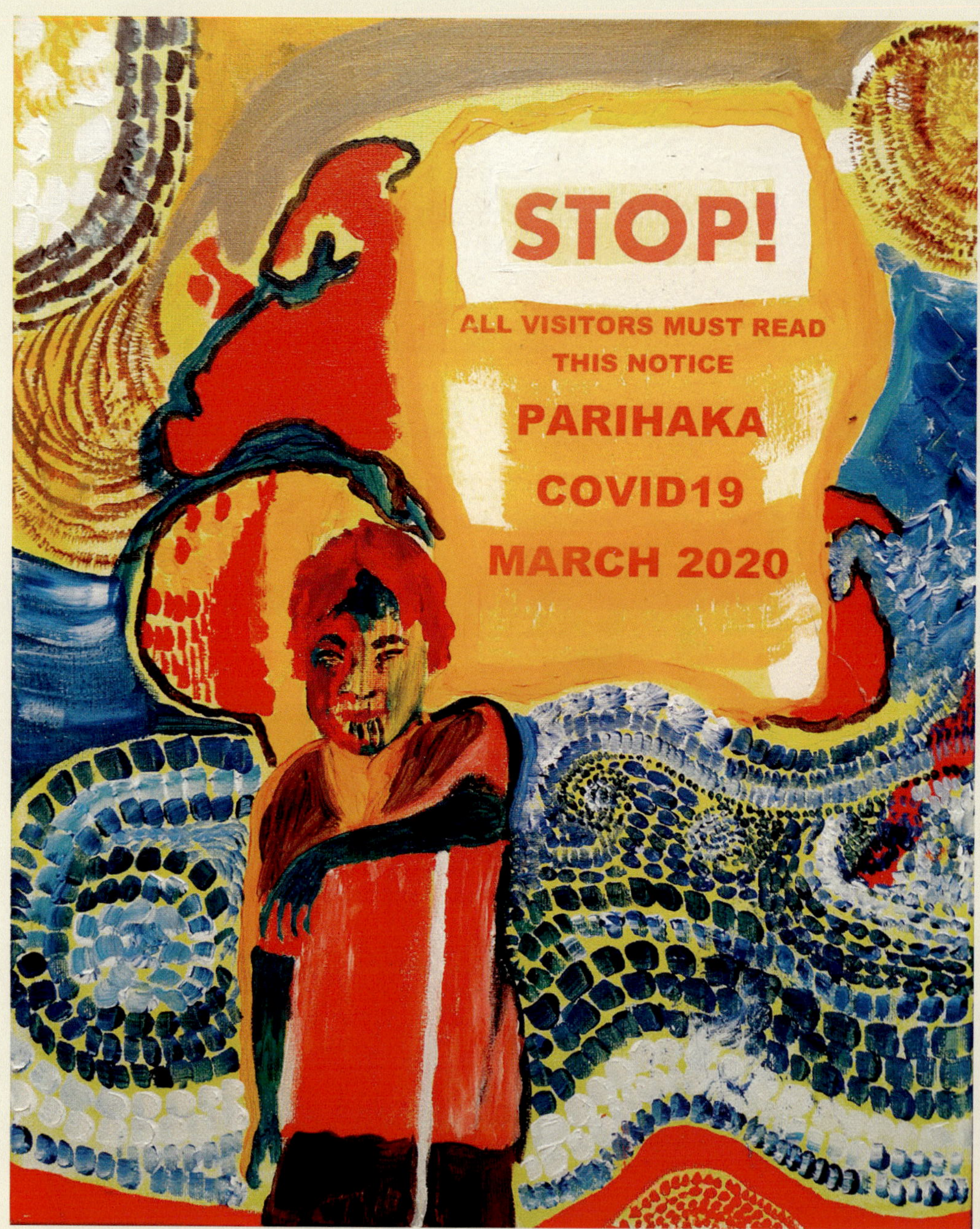

Plate 7. COVID roadblock sign painted by Maata Wharehoka

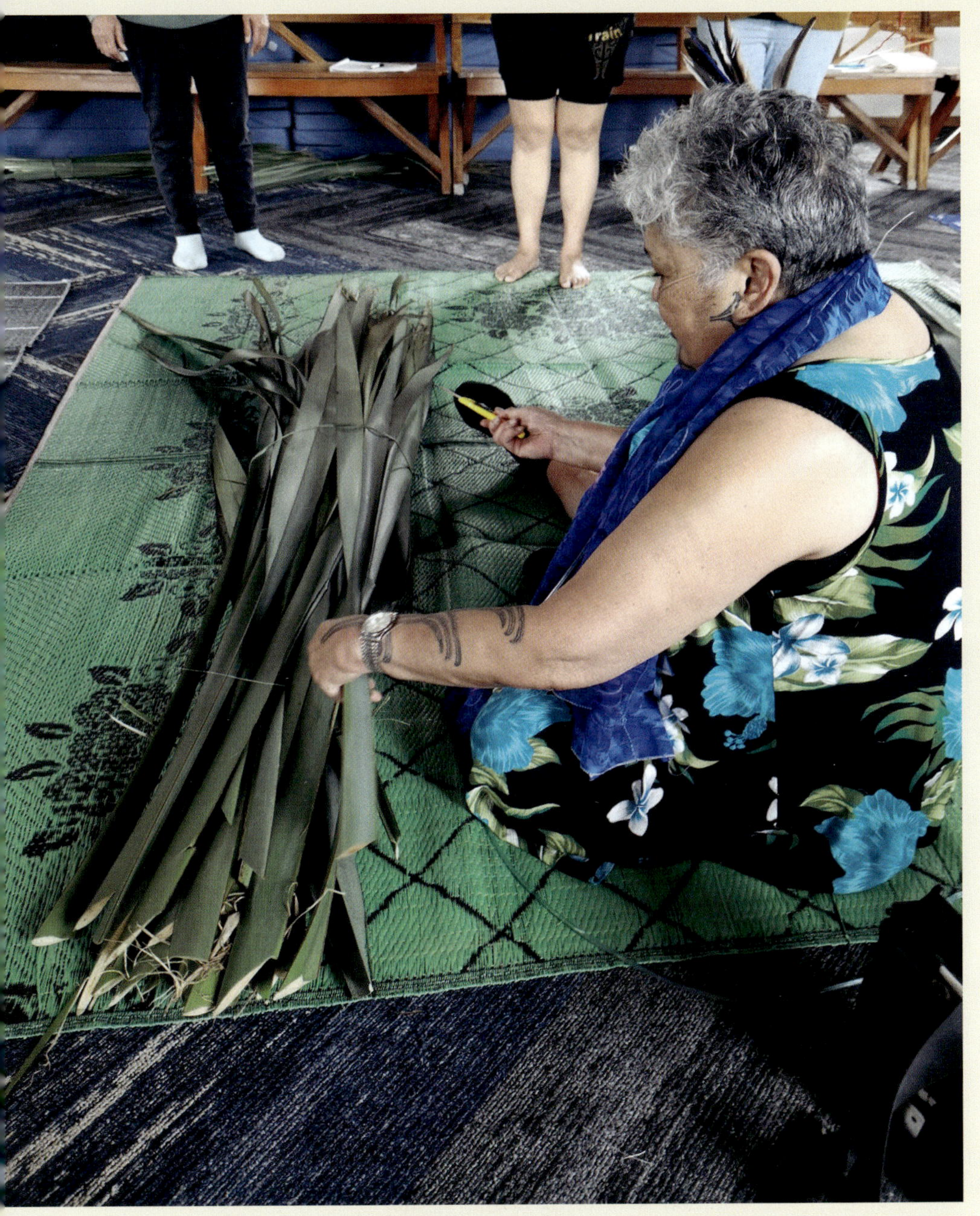

Plate 8. Maata stacking Harakeke for weaving
Photo by Jean Hikaka

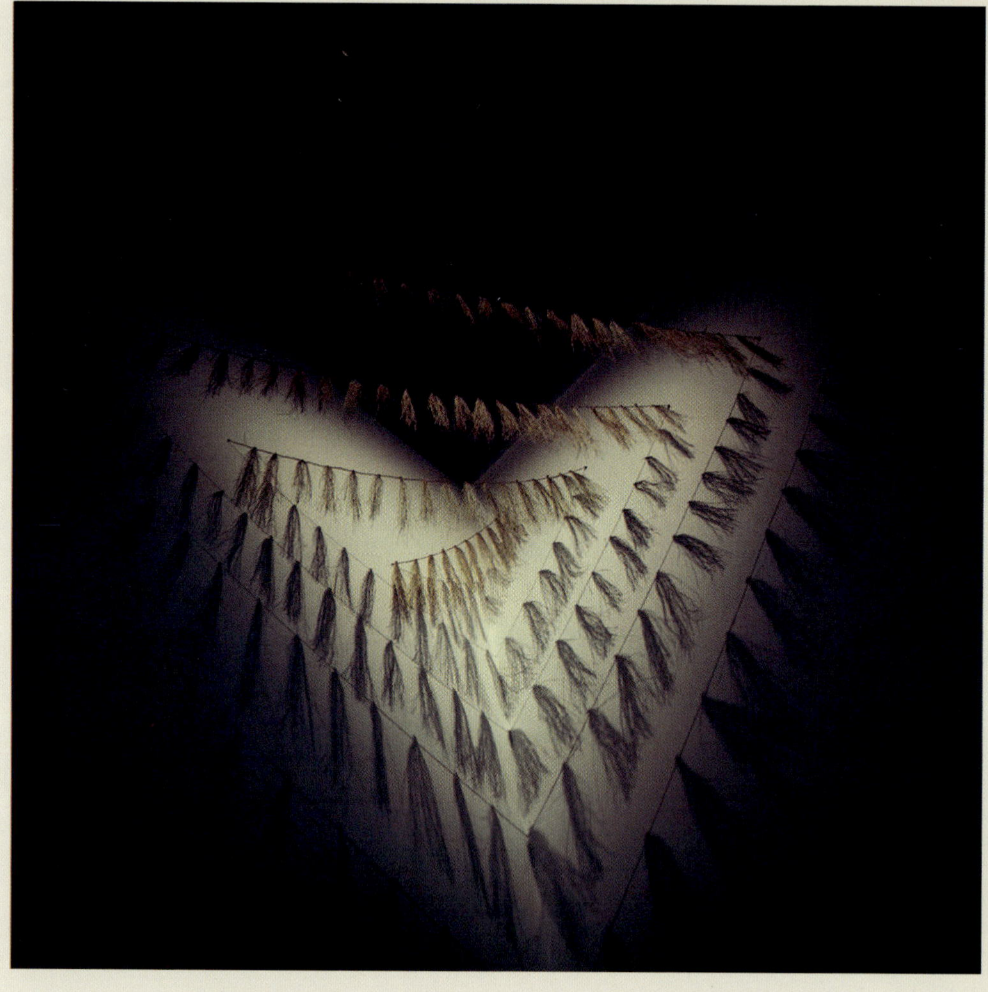

Plate 9. *Fibrous Soul* art by Maata Wharehoka
Photo by Jean Hikaka

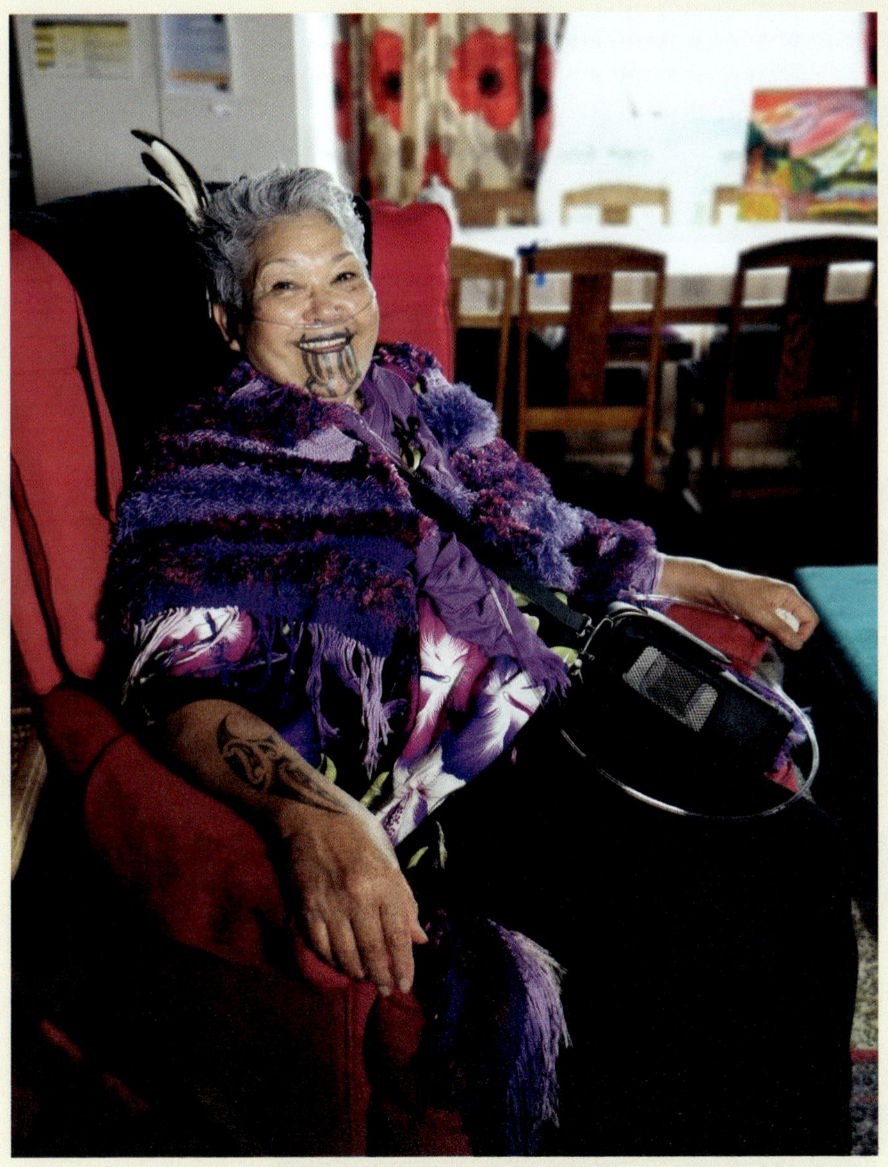

Plate 10. Maata in purple
Photo by Jean Hikaka

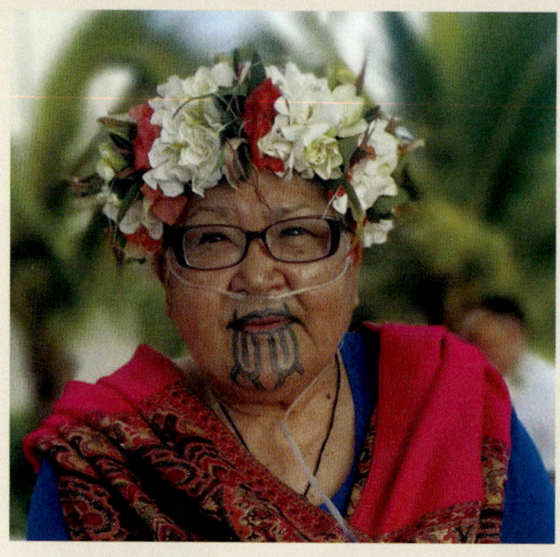

Plate 11. Maata with crown of flowers in Raratonga

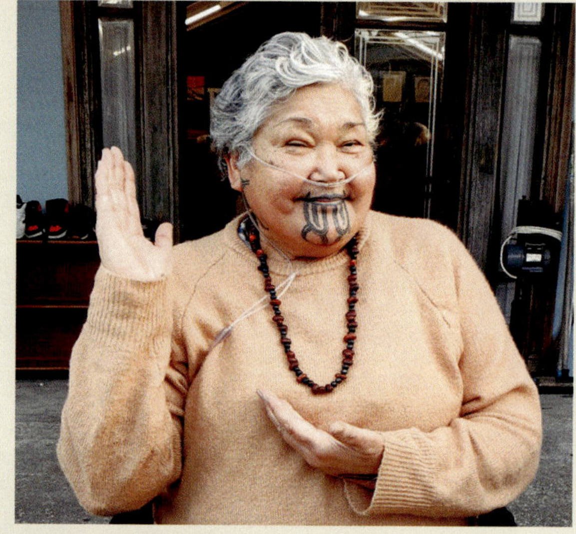

Plate 12. Maata Wharehoka outside her whare in Parihaka
Photo by Jean Hikaka

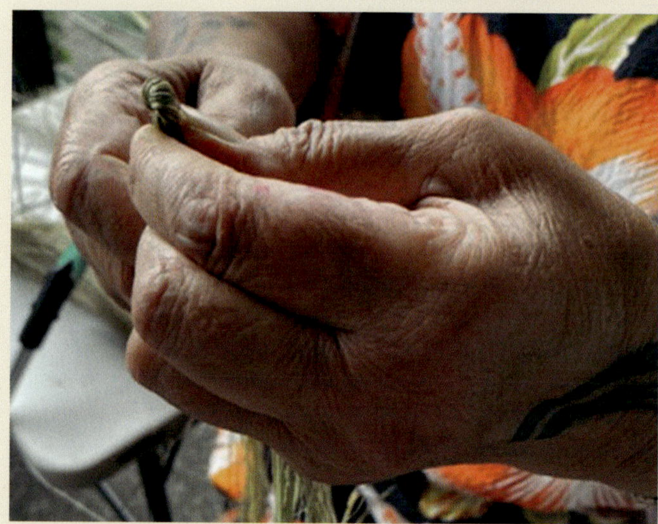

Plate 13. Maata's hands

Like Te Puea, the woman she identifies as one of her formative role models, Maata aims for real structural, systemic change and policy innovation. Imagine if cultural sensitivity was incorporated into how the COVID-19 pandemic, for instance, was managed throughout the world. While Jacinda Ardern, New Zealand's Prime Minister during the epidemic, was admired for her swift, definitive action to halt the spread of COVID in her country, she failed to include Māori communities or even to provide Te Reo versions of her broadcasts and directives. This forced Māori on marae to erect roadblocks in order to stop infection. In the US, similar conditions put Native Americans on reservations into a greater isolation than white people experienced. We need Indigenous women in policy-making positions for public health. Maata Wharehoka knows that and has advocated for it since she was a youth. She takes women's empowerment to another order of magnitude, and the world needs to know about her and follow her wisdom.

Women's Empowerment and Healthcare

Women's empowerment and healthcare have been linked since settlers arrived in New Zealand. They brought with them diseases of all kinds, physical, emotional, and spiritual, that ravaged Māori communities. The pre-European population for Māori was at least as high as 100,000, but by 1878 the census recorded 43,595 Māori. By 1896, this had slumped to 39,854. In 1874, the New Zealand Herald reported that "the race was dying." As of June 2023, the population has risen to 904,100, which is 17.3 percent of the national population (New Zealand government statistics). The rise is largely, if not completely, due to the efforts of women like Te Puea and the model of community health she innovated, and women like Maata who stand on her shoulders.

The largest smallpox epidemic recorded in New Zealand began in Whangarei in May 1913. It came into the country with a Mormon missionary from Arizona. He wanted to convert "the heathen." Smallpox spread furiously in Māori communities. There were 1777 Māori cases and 111 European. Te Puea immediately began creating open-air community health centers. They were outdoors because she had no funds to build enclosed shelters, but that did not stop her. She innovated a model of treating people close to their homes. She not only implemented the model in her region, she worked in community centers, and if there were none, she built them. It was an uphill struggle, but she never abandoned anyone. No one with smallpox died in the shelters she created (King 2006, 120–121).

Maata used this model in recommending that women be screened for cervical cancer where they live rather than making them come to hospital environments that they experience as unfriendly and even toxic. This is a model that should be in effect today, everywhere, and especially in Indigenous communities. Healthcare must be brought to the people, rather than asking people with little money and no transport to go to a place where they are disrespected and frequently ignored, and where there are no cultural comforts to ease their pain and anxiety.

Te Puea and Maata manifested a feminine model of compassionate, relational healthcare. As a healthcare provider, I am vociferous about this model. The correlation between regenerative, culturally sensitive healthcare and mortality is still marginalized, if not completely ignored. Women leaders repeatedly underscore it, pointing to the remedies, and then they are marginalized. But we are unstoppable. Our time is coming. Women in the healthcare field are rising up. Te Puea's vision, Maata's vision, and my vision of a healthcare system that is empowering to the recipients of it, is the healthcare of the future.

"Colonization is an attack on the soul," says Pania Te Whāiti, who developed a culturally sensitive counseling protocol for Māori women called Mai I Rangiātea (Te Whāiti et al. 1997, 85). Te Whāiti articulates what Maata Wharehoka lives in her relationships with the women she mentors, which is every woman who comes into contact with her. The underlying principle of Te Whāiti's approach is to declare to women that what they think and believe about themselves is far more important than what others think and believe about them. This is the credo that respected leaders like Tariana Turia, Whina Cooper, and Maata Wharehoka reiterate in their unprecedented campaigns, whether it is to stop the tobacco industry from manipulating people into suicidal smoking, restoring respect for Te Reo Māori and Māori rites of passage, or reclaiming land that was illegally confiscated and never ceded.

Maata's protocol for death and dying, Kahu Whakatere, is a stunning representation of her healthcare vision. Read more about Kahu Whakatere in the chapter on deathing in this book and also in the chapter on Māori art. Practices for death and dying, known as palliative care in the Western model, are frequently obscured as part of a larger effort to hide death and make it secretive. Māori culture is the polar opposite in its willingness to bring death and life together and out in the open.

Maata's leadership generates a potent feminine field. The women who came, for instance, to weave harakeke with her for an exhibit called Fibrous Soul in March 2024 in Taranaki, spoke of how their time together was a medicine circle that unified them, restoring their roots in the land. As one woman said, "I need to weave. It gives me strength. It helps me resolve the chaos of the world around me. It heals me from the illnesses that were brought here by Pākehā (Europeans). Weaving reminds me of who I really am. It is an honor to be called into this circle by Maata. It is her mana (sacred force) that calls me and that I heed."

Tiakitanga: Stewardship

While Māori were willing to adapt to Pākehā attire and were speedy learners and avid students of the Bible and the English language, Pākehā did not reciprocate by respecting Māori culture. The remarkable memories of Māori, as a by-product of oral learning, and the eloquence of Māori orators, along with the innate poetic lyricism of Te Reo Māori, were not lauded by Pākehā. Quite the reverse. Despite clear evidence of superior intelligence, adaptability, resilience, artistic mastery, and profound community cohesion, Pākehā continued to portray Māori as primitive. This is the universal phenomenon that has brought the world to metacrisis and the brink of apocalypse. If we can absorb the teachings and modeling of people like Maata Wharehoka and communities like Parihaka, we stand a chance of alchemizing our predicament into a world our children can safely inhabit.

Stewardship is implicit in all Māori practices and prioritized emphatically in birthing and deathing. See the chapters with those titles to understand the significance of beginning life and end-of-life rituals in terms of the bonding sense of belonging that unites all Māori, wherever they are in the world. Stewardship is innate in Māori women's leadership in all spheres of life, including parenting.

The way that Maata and her family have always lived is a reclamation of the respect due to a culture that hegemony, patriarchy, and colonization has consistently attempted to shred and discard, without success. Maata highlights the dignity and power of Māori women and the sanctity of motherhood and child-rearing. Birthing and deathing (Maata's coined word) are honored at Parihaka, the epic marae where Maata and her family live.

The oppressive forces of colonialism tore into the infrastructure of Māori life at every single level. It severed the people from each other, splintering and fragmenting the cohesive collective that made Māori communities so highly functional. This splitting apart of bonded units, and particularly the extended family nucleus, ravaged everyone. Practices of birthing and deathing were buried in shame and disrespect and, ultimately, obscurity. It was heartbreaking and soul crushing, but the ways in which Māori found resilience is a great tribute to them. We must pay attention to this rebound. All of us, regardless of culture, have been and continue to be colonized. Look at the reflections at the end of this and all chapters in this book for resources to decolonize your mind.

Marae are central to the continuity of Māori traditions, culture, and education. It is a classical institution that thankfully has been making a hearty resurgence. When you are welcomed onto the marae, or meeting grounds of the community, the first voice you hear is that of a woman. She is the kaikaranga, or communicator of the entire community. She symbolizes Papatūānuku, the earth mother, and Hine-nui-te-pō, the mother who embraces us at death. This shows the esteem women receive in Māori society.

As the kaikaranga, the communicator, of Parihaka, Maata sends a message to all Māori women, and to women generally, to hold that place of esteem with dignity, strength, and perseverance, no matter what else is happening. The ringing call of the pōwhiri (welcome) and the catalyzing movements of the haka pōwhiri (welcome ceremonial dance) encourage everyone within earshot to enter into the flow of resilient life that triumphs over adversity.

The Characteristics of Māori Wahine Leadership

Ehara taku toa i te takitahi, he toa takitini.
My success would not be bestowed on me alone, as it was not individual success, but success of a collective.

MĀORI WHAKATAUKĪ (PROVERB)

The leadership of Māori women is characterized by qualities that are instructive for all who aspire to leadership. Some of these include:

- Hūmārie (humility) that does not imply shyness, withholding or hesitancy. For instance, Maata Wharehoka is straightforward, direct, confrontational, even audacious, but she is, at the samc time, completely humble. Her humility comes from knowing her purpose and being dedicated to it. Maata teaches this to Māori wahine leaders: You are a vehicle of the needs of tangata whenua and their tūpuna. What your leadership requires is not about you; it is about your people.
- Honoring tikanga is essential for leadership. Māori women consult and embody tikanga (practices derived from Te Ao Māori, the Māori worldview).
- Guidance from tūpuna (ancestors). In Māori tikanga, there are prayers for almost every action. These prayers that precede everything invoke tūpuna so that they can guide all actions in the highest interest of tangata whenua, the people of the land.
- Weaving people together. Maata embodies this to perfection. I have never in my life seen anyone so artful in bringing together people from diverse backgrounds and regions with such a broad spectrum of skills and leading them into fruitful collaboration. In the meetings and events, like the Parihaka Peace Festivals that

Maata created, everyone found their role and purpose through her overseeing energy that was almost like an invisible net of emergent relationships. Maata delivers this mycorrhizal quality of Māori wahine leadership like the master weaver that she is.

- Connecting with people face-to-face is far superior to indirect communication. Whenever possible, deliver your leadership in person. Maata Wharehoka does this with every person she meets. Whoever is in her range is the recipient of her leadership. Whether she asks you to set the table or harvest harakeke, Maata is doing it with tikanga and her people in mind.
- Stewardship, tiakitanga, or kaitiakitanga is guardianship of the environment and the processes for protecting and caring for it. This is innate in Māori women's leadership. Remember the words of Rose Pere to Maata about healing Papatūānuku (Earth Mother)? See Maata's poem, "Stop Your Shit Dropping on Mother Papatuanuku"; it is a loud and clear transmission of this directive.

Pere the Rose
Oh, what a woman.
Yes, I agreed.
Of course, who would not?
Rose Pere my friend,
Feet stooped to mother earth,
Mind opened to father sky,
And the reality is rongo.
Rongo Māori
Rongo Wahine
Rongo

Rongoā for our earth

Rongoā for our whenua
Rongoā for our papa
Rongoā for our land.

Where doth it come?
Let the land soak
Beholden our land to those
Make well
Move the people to make well,
Make the place right.
Heal Papatūānuku.

Bring it on
People of people
Heal the land
Make well
Make good
Make sweetness happen.
Spread wellness.
Spread goodness.

Young to the old
Arm yourselves with the kupu
Freedom of mother earth
Stop polluting
Stop
Stop now!!!!

MAATA WHAREHOKA, APRIL 5, 2005

The rousing, straightforward words of Maata's poem demonstrate how these characteristics put Māori wahine leaders in a class of their own. It is an orientation toward leadership and facilitation that most of the world is unaware of, but that is nevertheless calling for our attention. Put these characteristics in the context of the leadership you know wherever you live and whatever groups you are part of or that you yourself facilitate. Is it not obvious that these characteristics would enhance leadership everywhere? One of the purposes of this book is to spread more widely the perspectives and values of Te Ao Māori. What most people do not know about Māori wahine reflects what they do not know about themselves or their capacities. It is time for that to change.

Women's Leadership and Self-Care

Maata once asked me to participate in a gathering she had created for women about self-care and healing. This was for women from throughout Aotearoa who were working for peace, for tangata whenua, with communities, and in the service professions. Women from throughout Aotearoa, of all ages, came together at Parihaka for this event. We experienced several of the healing arts, including dance and movement, weaving, singing, and art making. We learned to make poi, the light balls on strings of varying lengths that are twirled to accompany music and haka (fig. 6.1).

I was asked to describe healing from trauma and to conduct healing sessions for the community that gathered at Te Niho. This was a great honor. The entire experience, which lasted several days, demonstrated how Maata fulfills all the characteristics of Māori wahine leadership. She very deliberately created an environment where women who usually serve others could serve one another in a deeply feminine sanctuary of self-care. Te Niho, the marae that Maata caretakes, became like a nest house for women giving birth to themselves.

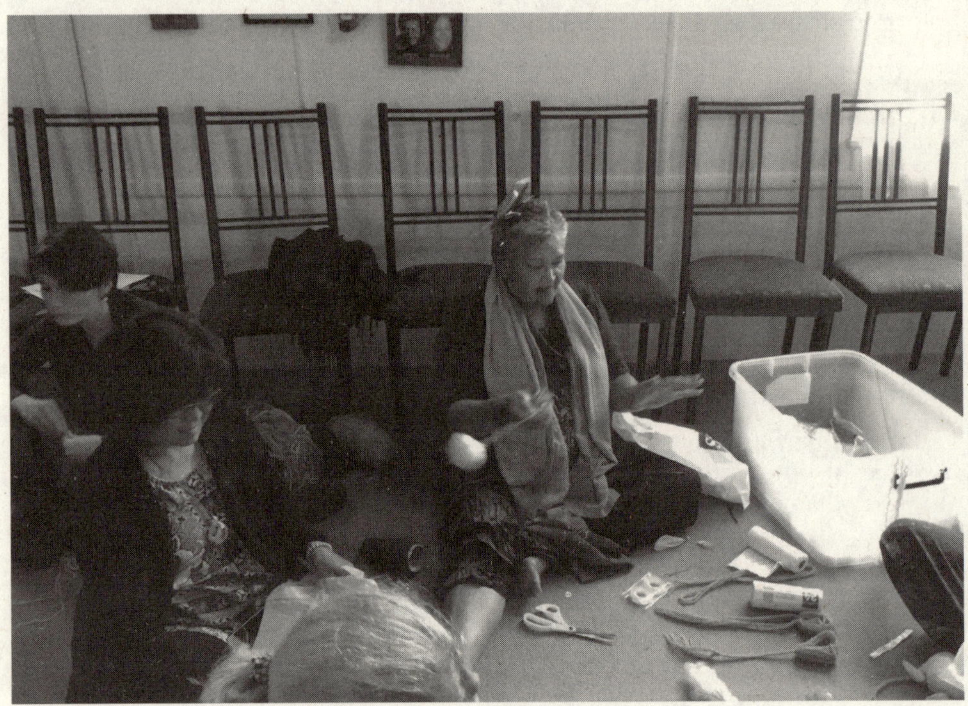

Fig. 6.1. Maata demonstrating poi

In doing this, Maata was also restoring herself. I have seen how brightly she shines when she is with other women, like those who come to weave with her. I believe it is accurate to generalize and say that those women who are devoted to tangata whenua are buoyed up by each other. Community is a reciprocal source of healing. It is the place of rest and hope. Women leaders are preeminently relational, and therefore they are healed in relationship with their peers, who recognize this need. The event in which Maata so graciously included me was just that. It reverberated with relational well-being under Maata's welcoming and inclusive guidance.

Events that Maata organizes always include kai, or meals. These are not just ordinary meals. They are meals made and served with

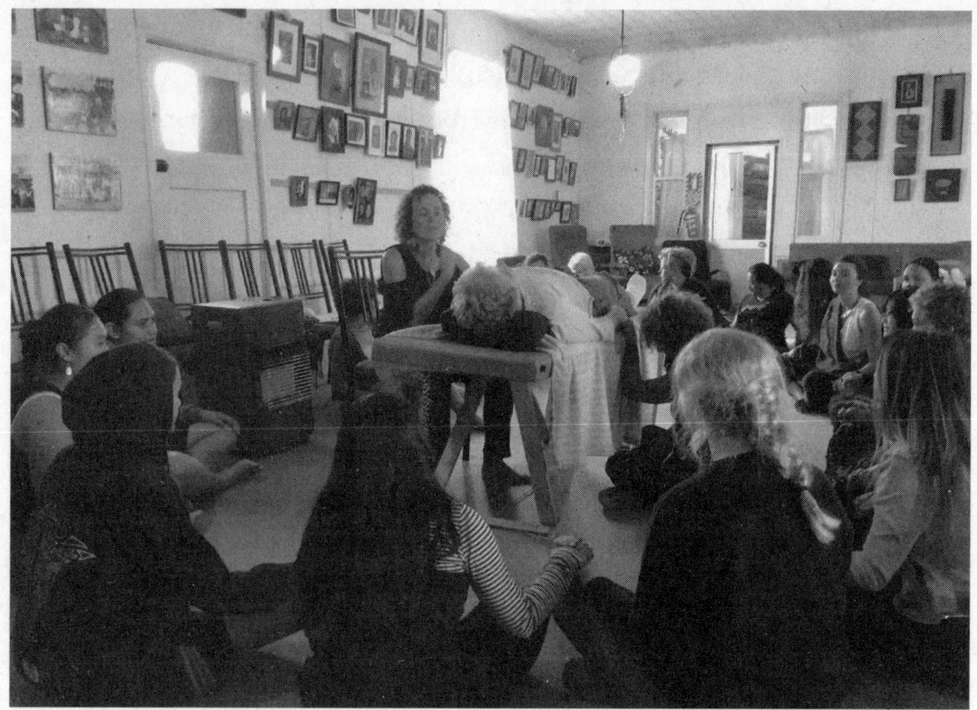

Fig. 6.2. Healing in community at Te Niho

care. In tikanga Māori, eating creates a transitionary segue from the sacred to the mundane. Maata relishes the food preparation as well as the consumption, particularly when it is in the company of friends and family. These shared meals are a source of restoration and joy for hard-working wahine, and Maata's events allow them to be nourished fully and beautifully. She makes sure that is the case.

Maata relishes beauty. You can see that in her choice of clothing, which is always colorful, and in how she adorns herself and her environment. Beauty restores her. When she visited me at my apartment in New Plymouth, where I was staying to be able to interview her, she sat for long stretches just gazing out the window at the sea, soaking up the healing of the ocean, restoring herself from all her mahi (efforts) in the service of others.

Maata loves music, and she loves to sing. In her quiet time, with family around, she might strum her ukelele, and her family members might join in with familiar songs from her era. Maata's cornucopia of service is emptied out over and over, but she can fill it easily and simply, in the company of her family and community, sharing meals, singing songs, and making art.

The concept of self-care is a modern one, probably not commonly known by kuia (women elders). I would like to suggest that the concept of kaitiakitanga, or stewardship, might also be applicable for kuia, who are the kaitiaki (guardians). Kuia, like Maata Wharehoka, deserve our manaakitanga, or gracious generosity in recognition of how they give their lives for tangata whenua.

REFLECTIONS ON HE WAHINE HE TAONGA— EVERY WOMAN IS A TREASURE

1. In your family and your community, what power do women's voices have? How does this sit with you?
2. What is your sense of the feminine perspective in your culture? How would you portray it?
3. How do you recognize colonization as an influence in terms of women's leadership?
4. What do you learn and how are you inspired by the leadership of Maata and the other women mentioned in this chapter, like Te Puea, in regard to healthcare and other systemic change?
5. Please describe how colonialism has disempowered the feminine perspective in your own life and lifetime, and the personal ramifications of that disempowerment.
6. What would you like to do to restore the voice of the feminine in your life, in your culture, in your community, and in the world?
7. How are elder women regarded in your family and in your community? Are they respected for their guardianship of life, or are they disregarded and made invisible? Please describe this reality and

how it impacts you, along with what you would like to do about it.

8. If you are a woman, and if you are a leader, what have you learned about self-care and leadership?
9. Is stewardship of our environment, of our world in crisis, a characteristic of leadership for all those in charge? If so, how do you enforce this—by requiring it of yourself as a leader and of the leaders you endorse?

7
Whakaora: Restoring Health

We need to heal the ways we think, feel, relate, exchange, and exist. The only possible answer is healing as a collective body.

Maria Jara Qquerar, Quechua Maestra

In her watershed treatise on decolonizing medicine, *Inflamed*, Dr. Rupa Marya and Raj Patel (2021, 24) say, "Practitioners of modern medicine are not trained to be healers. They are trained to be biomedical technicians." Maata Wharehoka trained herself to be a healer. Her intimate knowledge of the healthcare needs of her people and the ways in which every aspect of their well-being has been attacked by colonialism was evident when she was only fourteen years old and won the distinguished St. John's Grand Prior's Award for exemplary service in healthcare. It seemed a direct line to her becoming a public health nurse. Maata modeled culturally sensitive healthcare before that terminology was even used. Holism is innate in her. She has never lost sight of the power of Māori advocating for and shaping Māori healthcare. She has been doing it since she was a teenager!

Dr. Marya, a physician schooled in the United States, continues, "Doctors are trained not only to look exclusively at the patient as a solitary individual—shorn of context or structure, stripped of life in all its complexity—but to treat that individual as a broken machine, as a dysfunctional and occasionally noncompliant robot bearing a symptom." Rongoā, Māori medicine, is the polar opposite. It embraces the whole person, including their history and their physical environment. Maata's culturally sensitive, holistic, and nature-attuned approach to healthcare is what the world is desperate for right now. The climate crisis has made this yearning a regular headline.

Healthcare around the world has failed Indigenous people. In truth, it has failed all people, but the insult to Indigenous people is most reprehensible. Just as European settlers in Aotearoa sought to erase traditional Māori medicine, Western medicine throughout the world tends today to disregard, minimize, insult, and ridicule folk and ancient healing wisdom. That is starting to shift as the scientifically sound underpinnings of these resources are acknowledged and integrated into medical practice. The way in which Jean Hikaka and her mother, Maata Wharehoka, were able, in Taranaki, to introduce traditional Māori methods for tying the umbilical cord of the newborn baby is an example of this shift. See the birthing chapter in this book for this healing story.

The New Zealand Ministry of Health (2024, 1) reports that Māori are disproportionately affected by chronic disease, including mental health conditions, and experience a higher burden of anxiety, depression, and mental distress compared to non-Māori. Māori women are twice as likely as non-Māori women to be diagnosed with cervical cancer and 2.5 times more likely to die from the disease. Regular cervical screening can reduce a woman's risk of developing cancer by 90 percent. Nevertheless, Māori women are reluctant to have screenings in an environment that is unfamiliar and even disrespectful of their lifestyle.

Knowing this, Maata Wharehoka introduced radical changes to healthcare by recommending that screenings could happen on the marae, that easy-going conversation and even food should be included in the screening environment whether in a hospital, at home, on the marae, or elsewhere. As a result of her effective outreach, screening rates increased substantially. In this way, Maata Wharehoka pioneers culturally sensitive healthcare to this very day.

True healing is only possible when it is culturally sensitive. Maata has always known this. She is my mentor in this regard, as I have launched a global program called "Regenerative Health for A Climate Changing World" that is based on reskilling medicine via cultural sensitivity. Maata's model was Te Puea Herangi's, who, even though she was not trained to be a nurse as Maata was, was still able to look at Māori health needs and healthcare delivery systems from both Māori and Pākehā perspectives. That is what is necessary for systemic change. How Te Puea acted on behalf of her people during the deadly influenza and smallpox pandemics in the mid-1900s, when Māori communities were underserved, even abandoned, and without resources, remains a model for healthcare today, particularly in regard to compassionate service for Indigenous communities. See the chapter in this book on women's empowerment, "He Wahine He Taonga: Every Woman Is a Treasure," for more about Te Puea and her healthcare activism strategies.

Parihaka met the challenge of the COVID pandemic like a strong, regenerative health savvy community, protecting its members and keeping out threats. Maata utilized her skills as a public health nurse in the interest of her community and her whānau. She also used her artistry. Because Parihaka was vulnerable as a tourist site, and because there was a unified commitment to keep infection out, roadblocks and gates were erected to prevent the entry of people who might be carrying COVID. Maata contributed bright and beautiful signs with the clear message to keep out, stay away, stop, do not enter (see plate 7). Everything Maata does is beautiful, even if she is saying, "No way. Stay out!"

Maata knows from her personal experience that art is healing. Her paintings, weavings, and poetry in this book demonstrate how art lifts her up, allows her to voice her truth, and is an outlet for her passionate love and dedication. When Rose Pere instructed Maata to "heal Papatūānuku," she was speaking of healthcare at its source. Maata knows, and frequently declares, that everything she does is designed for healing. She fulfills the true definition of what it means to implement healthcare.

The Root Structure of Health: Te Ao Māori Meets Attachment Theory

I have lived most of my life with the certainty that I was poorly attached. How could it be otherwise, I wondered, particularly after I became a neuropsychologist. In the literature I read by every highly respected author, from Winnicott to Mate, from Mahler to Schore, it was unquestionable that, given the violence in my home, given the sexual abuse and dysfunction of my family, I had to be poorly attached. That was certainly what was wrong with me. This was why I struggled with relationships. This was why I had so much difficulty with confidence. The grief of how I was so marked by my family's dysfunction was endless. It was a bottomless well.

It is only recently that I pierced the lie of this assumption and its colonial, patriarchal underpinnings. It has become crystal clear to me that, in fact, the opposite is true. I am amazingly, brilliantly attached and bonded to what really matters—which is the natural world, creativity, and my lineage. Not only that, but I am incredibly resilient in adapting that attachment, those bonds and connections, to a variety of ecosystems and communities. It is not case dependent. It is within me and inseparable from me. Indeed, I have been powerfully and securely attached from the moment I took form. This is a matriversal understanding. It comes from the standpoint of being akin to the natural world. It is also the perspective of an embryologist who understands human development from the beginning of life.

I attribute this awakening, in part, to my time in Aotearoa with people like Rangatira Maata Wharehoka and her family. They did not impart the awareness directly. It grew as a by-product of my time with them and my capacity to track what was being aroused in me as a result of being in that environment and with the Māori people.

The Indigenous worldview that Maata and her family embody communicated itself in daily actions, not in lectures, discourse, or books. This is matriversal education. As I harvested flax with them for weaving, ate with them, laughed and cried with them, something that had always been with me surfaced from where it was buried under the misogynistic, elitist psychology required for mental health professionals. The ease with which Kuia (Elder) Maata could shed what was untrue reminded me of what was natural to me, but what I had been taught to be ashamed of or suppress. She inspired me to prioritize my own experience over the dictates of academia, which is, for the most part, disembodied. Maata had no need to pamper or indulge anything untrue.

What surfaced as a result of this communion with Maata and others at the epic Parihaka marae in Taranaki, was me, the real me, the one who had always been deeply connected to everything and everyone. It is actually because of my deeply connected, compassionate awareness that I am able to develop my creativity and my intelligence, even when my ideas are not necessarily popular, and even if they are ridiculed. Nothing stops Maata from voicing her truth because her sense of herself is too deeply rooted. She knows that her tūpuna (ancestors) have her back. She mirrored this for me, and the reflection stuck.

I had previously been convinced that I was an outcast, an oddity, but this, I discovered, was imposed upon me. It did not arise from within me. It had never been true. That became clear to me at Parihaka, in the company of Maata Wharehoka. I cannot overemphasize the magnitude of the about-face that comes with the somatic realization of belonging. I was never outcast. No one is. I am welcomed in by the universe, celebrated, desired, and loved. The cell-deep certainty of this changed everything.

I have always been deeply bonded with the spirit world, though I had no language for claiming that before. In Maata's environment, the spirit world sits down for kai (food) along with everyone else. It was that unerasable, sustaining bond that was a natural part of everyday, practical activity that came home to me. I saw that I had always had this bond and that it had allowed me to transcend the cruelty and chaos of a family home riddled with unresolved trauma. Maata and her family have worked hard to reclaim their language and their tikanga (practices), often adapting them to current conditions, with great success, like *Kahu Whakatere*, the practices for death, dying and burial. This is a teaching for the world.

Even in a third-story tenement walk-up in the Bronx where I was born, I had access to the natural world. I was a stargazer. The night sky was my land. The constellations and the planets, the wind and the clouds, were my friends. I was not escaping. I was bonding and attaching to my kin, and I was smart enough to keep that private. I know this is true in my flesh, in my very cells, which most academics do not see as validation of knowledge. Thanks to Maata's modeling, I no longer care what academics or anyone think about what I know to be true.

I was taught to discount myself by a system that is unconscious of Indigenous ways of knowing. For that patriarchal, colonial system, inner knowing, particularly when it does not accord with patterns documented in texts and diagnostic manuals, is silenced and often judged as pathology. I can remember, distinctly, when a noted trauma authority who I was working closely with responded to my comment that the trauma in my life began in utero by shaking his head in disbelief and redirecting the conversation. I was domesticated to obediently go along with that. Until now.

Embracing the truth that I have always harbored an unquestionable sense of belonging, that I am united with the natural world in ways that allow me to merge with it, has changed everything for me. Maata and other Indigenous people have survived because of this knowing. So have I. Can you see how Te Ao Māori, the Māori worldview, and particularly the standard bearing of women like Kuia Maata Wharehoka, is leadership for a world in crisis, a world that needs an Indigenous and a matriversal perspective?

From the moment that I began to write, which started around seven or eight years old, I was reclaiming my language. Language is identity. My true identity is in the language of my writing. It is a poetic dialect, like Te Reo Māori. I continue to be dedicated to reclaiming my own language. This is a continuum.

For decades, Māori were punished, often severely beaten, for speaking their own language, Te Reo. That pain reverberates through generations. Te Reo is an exquisite, metaphoric, generative, and flexible language. As a people who learned and shared knowledge through oral transmission, the theft of language was excruciating. Yet, today, Māori are in the process of recovering their language. Māori waiata (songs) echo in meeting halls, on sports fields, on the internet, on radio and television, at churches, social events, in gymnasiums, schools, and festivals. The singers smile broadly as they belt out the songs that they all know by heart. Their joy is contagious. The spirit of reclamation through polyvocality has begun to triumph over the losses. Voicing truth in one's own language brings health.

A similar reclamation is happening in other places where language has been stolen, including for me and for women globally, especially Indigenous women, as we rise. The language of our original brilliance was stolen from us, but it is still alive, and we are finding exactly where it was hidden within us. This will root our secure attachment to what is real and help us recover from decades of living in shock from the theft of our heart-and-soul language. It is liberating to see the ways in which the matriversal perspective parallels and is intertwined with an Indigenous worldview through a collective reclamation of language.

REFLECTIONS ON WHAKAORA: CULTURALLY SENSITIVE HEALTHCARE

1. How do you evaluate the healthcare system and its delivery of resources in your region? Do you feel that it is culturally sensitive? Do you consider it effective? Describe how it is or is not.
2. The idea, and the practice, of providing healthcare for people in the language they are comfortable with and honoring their cultural mores for receiving healthcare seems to be common sense, but it is largely absent in modern healthcare. Can you consider how effectiveness is diminished when healthcare disregards cultural requirements? Imagine if your own culture was valued in the healthcare you receive. What would that look like for you, for your family, and for your community?
3. An Indigenous view of healthcare is holistic. It includes deep listening and the recognition of environmental and epigenetic influences on health. It is also family centered, always taking the collective into consideration as an aspect of health. It incorporates kinship and resources of the natural world as medicine. The absence of these values is highlighted now as climate anxiety shapes mental and

emotional well-being and erodes health generally in unprecedented and unpredictable ways. With a knowledge of the Indigenous worldview, how would you like to see healthcare evolve?

4. Can you see how a health challenge you or a family member has faced recently could be reframed from a culturally sensitive vantage point? What would that look like? What would that feel like?
5. What happens in your consciousness when you take attachment theory beyond the nuclear family and see it as being inclusive of the natural world, seen and unseen, animals, plants, and even ideas? Describe how this paradigm change could shift your relationship to yourself and your health.
6. Can you put yourself in the center of your own healthcare and the healthcare of your family and your community? In other words, what happens to your view of health when you see it without reliance on an authority structure? What would change in your life and in the life of your family if you lived as the center of your own healthcare? Look at how Parihaka took responsibility for itself during the COVID pandemic. Is this a model you could or would replicate? How?
7. What is your sense of the correlation between language and health? Are you free to voice your truth? If you are, can you track how this expands your experience in the world and how that expansion equates with health?
8. If you have ever had your voice squelched or suffocated, what impact did you notice on your well-being? Do these reflections allow you to have more understanding and compassion for the struggle to reclaim one's true language?

8

Deathing

Kahu Whakatere

Just a few months before this book was finalized, Maata Wharehoka transitioned out of her body. Her dedication to restoring the tikanga (sacred practices) of Kahu Whakatere—the ceremonies of dying, death and burial—came full circle as she knew they would. Every member of her family and wider circle of friends knew exactly what to do to honor her. This adds considerable significance to this chapter.

Maata had frequently predicted her death because her health was so severely undermined that everything was difficult for her. Yet she still glowed with a radiance that belied those predictions. Her actual death, therefore, came as a shock. Even in death, Maata Wharehoka was indomitable and in charge. She is the Queen of Peace, now and forever.

Te Pō Whakamutunga—The Final Night

Through the creation and practice of Kahu Whakatere, a ritual to embrace bereavement, transition, and loss, Maata Wharehoka has made it possible for death to be a peacemaker and unifier. Kahu

Whakatere redefines the meaning of death and creates what Maata calls "deathing" as a parallel to "birthing."

Kahu Whakatere restores the traditional Māori view of death and dying, but it also goes beyond that. It integrates death into life and contributes to it, while simultaneously functioning as an enactment of reconciliation, acceptance, and authentic grieving. Kahu Whakatere empowers families to engage directly with their loved ones as they pass from the physical plane and to honor their lives as they resolve any tensions or obstacles to expressing their love. This expands deathing into peacemaking.

In delivering and standing boldly for Kahu Whakatere as a rite of passage, Maata is a force for reconnection and cultural sovereignty. The process is compelling and attractive because of its authenticity. Kahu Whakatere is in bold contrast to the detached, formulaic undertaking and funeral processes. It returns warmth, vibrancy, and kinship into the journeys of grief, loss, and transition from the body.

In describing how Kahu Whakatere helped them in the loss of their mothers, two women I spoke with became radiant. Their eyes brightened with tears and also with joy, as they relayed how honored they were to be guided to orchestrate the passages of their beloved family members using the sanctuary of the Kahu Whakatere ceremony. The death garments and mats woven by family members added natural, sustainable, and aesthetic beauty. They also imparted for everyone a living methodology and a structured physical process through which their grief was digested, assimilated, and metabolized. Family members, community, and friends went beyond loss to peace. They played their instruments in the orchestra of Kahu Whakatere.

Those who experience Kahu Whakatere become so enthralled with its beneficial choreography that they want to learn how to share it with other families. It is a gift to every cherished elder.

Thus, a legacy has been reborn for a people through the diligence of Maata Wharehoka. Demonstrating how it is possible to turn away from the Eurocentric practices imposed on Māori and instead successfully enact culturally relevant rituals at the end stage of life has been a breakthrough. Everyone who participates in Kahu Whakatere is uplifted. This is how death becomes life. This is how death, birth, and legacy are interwoven.

Kahu means amniotic sac, or caul, in Te Reo Māori. It is the word for what embraces, protects, and envelopes the embryo that travels through the womb to the world of light, the earth plane. It also refers to the woven garment that clothes the deceased in the ritual of Kahu Whakatere. This garment, woven by the family and friends of the departed, contains all the emotions they have sorted in letting go, so that the one who has died can securely, fearlessly set off in the boat of death to another dimension. Whakatere means to navigate, so Kahu Whakatere is the sac of navigation, the woven vehicle and protective shield of a joyous, love-filled, and honorable farewell.

Māori were stripped of their sustaining rituals through colonization, and Maata has turned this around as the champion of cultural restoration and agency in life and death. Not only has she created and disseminated the regenerated process of dying through Kahu Whakatere, she also champions the individual right to choose the moment of death.

After a devastating car accident, Maata's respiratory system suffered so severely that she was not able to get the oxygen she needs without support. More than once she has come back from the dead. But she lives in pain and discomfort and wants to be able to determine when she has had enough. Because of this, Maata advocated for euthanasia legislation in Aotearoa New Zealand, and that initiative succeeded. Maata says it makes her happy to know that she can make this choice for herself. From the viewpoint of some, this position challenges tikanga, but Maata's understanding is that euthanasia is a legitimate evolution of tikanga Māori about death, just as Kahu Whakatere evolves the original rituals for death and dying.

The weaving and other arts of Kahu Whakatere are so stunning that Govett-Brewster, the major museum and art gallery in New Plymouth, the largest metropolitan area closest to Parihaka, hosted an exhibit to feature it. The beauty of the mats and the cloak that envelops the body of the deceased imparts spiritual strength and awe. The sustainability of all the materials speaks volumes about Māori culture, which honors and protects the earth in all its manifestations.

Each step in the Kahu Whakatere experience reignites the cellular memory of the connections all participants have to a lineage of wisdom. This happens simultaneously with revitalizing their relationship with the departed, just as they are letting go. The dying person is held securely in the loving embrace of lineage, knowing that they are entering another realm of their family, their ancestral bond. Both mourners and the deceased are linked by their personal and collective bond to a timeless stream of belonging and purpose. This healing brings the marae to the community, even if the ceremony does not physically occur on a marae. Marae is a state of consciousness, as well as a location.

The marae is the place where you do all the healing.

Maata Wharehoka

Death as Evolution

Kahu Whakatere is active. Every person has a role to play. The body is washed and dressed by family members with the prescribed herbs that they gather. The garment that covers the body is woven by family and friends as well as the mat upon which the body is placed. Love and connection are everywhere in the Kahu Whakatere practice.

Healing conversations accompany the harvesting and the weaving and all the activity leading to the actual burial or tangihanga. Maata and others she has trained guide and assist the family in their active participation in every step of the process. Everyone is evolving, including the one who is dying or has passed. Younger family members witness and play a role so that death and dying is not to be feared. It is familiar. It is human. Death is life.

Contrast this with the funeral and burial industry that substitutes connection with separation. In the European model death is isolated from life. The body is treated for burial by strangers away from the family, behind closed doors. Children are kept away and therefore fear death and dying. In my practice as a trauma therapist, I listened to countless stories about family losses in which my client, now an adult, was not informed or included or involved in any way with the passing of a sibling or a grandparent, or anyone who was part of the family, even a close family friend. As a result, people feel haunted by the loss, unresolved, because they were not given the opportunity to grieve. It was assumed that children should be "protected" from loss when, in fact, excluding them made them vulnerable unnecessarily, often to decades of confusion.

Researchers in the fields of palliative care and thanatology name loneliness and the fear of death, and specifically of not being remembered, not being recognized as valuable, as prevalent throughout Western culture (Sawyer 2024; Rezapour 2022; Ellis et al. 2012). The constructs of Kahu Whakatere, borne out of Maata's passionate intensity to heal her people, are antidotes to these widespread and crucifying anxieties. Everyone would benefit from the principles of Kahu Whakatere.

People who have a history of not being able to express their fear of death, or who are without partners, relatives, or friends with whom they have strong bonds and a sense of true intimacy, experience what palliative care providers call "disintegrative deaths." As they approach death, whether in a hospital bed or at home, with hospice care, these lonely people suffer with an ontological discord because they are partitioned from the rest of life, from the human community that is everyone's birthright (Sinclair 2011, 182). Kahu Whakatere restores that birthright.

The underpinnings of Kahu Whakatere offer a way toward death as integrated evolution, with the confidence that dying is natural and that you are welcomed beyond death just as you are meant to be welcomed at birth. This is why Maata chose the word *deathing* for the Kahu Whakatere process. She equates death, from her direct experience with the death of her sister, her husband, and with her own life-threatening moments, as well as her experience as a mother delivering her children, and as a woman who lost babies in childbirth, with birthing. This guidance from an Indigenous woman, from a kuia, an elder, speaks to this moment in history, when death is everywhere. Our entire civilization is on the brink of death. The guidance of Kahu Whakatere could lead us away from that precipice by bringing us together to honor life, including all that is dying.

Tūpuna/Ancestors

He Tūpuna, he mokopuna.
We are all ancestors; we are all grandchildren.

Māori Whakataukī (Proverb)

The one who is dying is spiritually aligned, often hearing and seeing their ancestors, and they are simultaneously as innocent and receptive as a child or grandchild. The veils are lifted and commune as death comes closer. The structures of Kahu Whakatere actively encourage tūpuna to come to this communion. In Western culture, this could be pathologized, patronized, and pushed aside. Maata's deathing process reinvigorates the natural process of communion with the spirits that come closer and closer as one lies dying.

Tūpuna are as integral to Kahu Whakatere and the dying process as those still in their bodies. They arrive to provide guidance and comfort. The one who is dying needs, craves, and reaches for this accompaniment. Whānau (family) share tūpuna, so it is only right that they should all gather together in the safe, sacred, and familiar place of the tangihanga (gathering to say farewell to the deceased or mourning ceremony).

Just as there is a belief in the safety of birthing at home, so is there a comfort in deathing at home. Tūpuna and mokopuna are the headlights on the undying vehicle of Māori culture. That is why they are so completely integral to Kahu Whakatere.

As a mother and grandmother, myself, I have been awed and deeply touched by the sacred law of honoring tūpuna and elders in Māori families. We will all grow old and approach the moment of death with some trepidation. How sweet to have the ritual of Kahu Whakatere awaiting us, giving us the security of being wrapped, held, contained, guided, supported, loved, and cherished by and with our loved ones on the earth and our loved ones who await our reunion.

Kahu Whakatere

The room is brimming with a co-emergent blend of focus and concentration, mixed with the chatter of people who feel safe in their fond connection with one another. Elders are ushered into the space and gently moved toward comfortable, pillowed places. They easily begin sharing in the tender grieving and honoring of the one who has departed this realm of consciousness.

Children play on the periphery, free to make their sounds and be themselves. The environment is soft and thoroughly, utterly human. The hum of talk is like a collective song of life, though it is death that has brought everyone together. Women assemble bouquets of herbs, their work-worn hands fluttering with a task they know well. Family members sit close to the body of the loved one who has passed. The deceased, as if in a serene sleep, is fully integrated into this gathering, not separate from it.

The mat on which the body rests has been woven by some of the people in the room. The deceased is elegantly clothed, and preserved by the kinds of herbs the women are bundling. The room is redolent with the scent of those herbs and the harakeke of the mats. Undulating waves of singing drift through everything in this sacred space, along with crying, and occasional wailing. Some may be chuckling at fond memories with their beloved friend or family member. People walk over to the deceased and touch the hands or the face, speaking softly, whispering confidences. They might even tell a joke that they know the deceased would enjoy.

At a prescribed time, the Kahu Whakatere participants move outside and follow the pallbearers carrying the body to the marae urupā (cemetery). Dances and prayers accompany them. There is unquestionable sadness and loss, but there is also unbroken, spirited continuity. The air is crisp, and the sun is bright. The surrounding Pohutukawa trees scatter their needle-like red strands as if making an offering. The body is carried on a structure made by hand from the natural wood available, and rests on a beautiful woven mat. All these items are derived from sustainable materials, harvested, softened, and woven or built by the community. The burial is a group endeavor. Every aspect of the process is intimate, connected to the deceased, and in attuned service to the entire family and their collective extended family. Friends as well as kin join together in unconditional unity. The presence of the tūpuna, the ancestors of the deceased, is palpable.

After the burial, no one leaves. Everyone remains together to share a sumptuous meal, thereby defining the boundary between the sacredness of what they have shared and the return to a more ordinary agenda. Tikanga Māori is astute in providing these boundaries and definitions. What is sacred? What is mundane? How do we differentiate them? Being able to make these discernments gives structure to life and clarity to transitions. It is correct and safe to separate from the deceased, knowing they are protected. There is no guilt in celebrating the wonderful food and company of those on the earthly plane. In this way tikanga Māori is psychologically and emotionally supportive of everyone in the sphere of the deceased, particularly the nuclear family. Death is integrated into life, and these are the steps to help you to feel that integration.

Maata Wharehoka knows birth and death. She knows what it means to carry and deliver babies, and she knows what it feels like to bury them. She knows how to welcome life and to steward it, and she knows how to say goodbye. She is also intimate with the tūpuna, the unseen realms and ancestral forces, that accompany every stage of life. Maata is never alone in her wisdom. Even as I write these words for you, Maata Wharehoka is communing with her tūpuna.

In Māori culture no one is alone. This is perhaps the primary teaching for these times, and it seems appropriate that it should come through Kahu Whakatere, the design that Maata has reinvented from tikanga Māori for deathing, here and now. In the United States, where I live, many people die alone.

Elderly die in shabby, solitary rooms. The poor who are ill suffer and die without sanctuary. Hegemonic culture abandons those without financial capacity. It is a culture solely for the young and wealthy. Everyone else is disappeared. Let us learn from Kahu Whakatere about the communion and comfort of sharing death as a natural transition that assembles with tenderness, respect, and communion, all that life has offered for each and every precious being. Everyone has a family. That is what the tūpuna say.

REFLECTIONS ON DEATHING

As we reflect on Maata's teachings about death, encapsulated in the living process of Kahu Whakatere, we have an opportunity to not only authentically honor Māori culture but to also bring its gifts into our lives, our communities, and the organizations we are serving. Maata dares to challenge dominant culture premises and to manifest alternatives that touch on the true needs of humanity. Ask yourself the questions below as you consider following Maata's model of voicing truth and acting courageously from a deep love for your people, for humanity, and a commitment to restoring innate belonging, unity, and multicultural alignment in life and in death.

1. How do I want to experience my passing from this body?
2. How do I want to be remembered?
3. What and who are the individuals and communities I want to accompany me through my dying process?
4. Are there cultural traditions from my ancestors that I want included in my death and dying process?
5. How can I build the container I need to die in an integrated, peaceful way?
6. How can I share a fearless and welcoming approach to death with my family and the communities in which I participate?
7. What can I learn about my ancestors so that I can consciously join

them in my dying process and invite them to guide and support me as I journey toward them?

8. How can I honorably share with others the lineage and practices of Kahu Whakatere as a source of inspiration for integrated death and dying, and for cultural reclamation?

CONCLUSION

A New Life

It has always been about the children of the future. All the sacrifice and the healing from the core wounds of colonization, all the learning and the organizing of programs and networking. All the educational outreach, and the effort to be of service, all of it has been done in the name of the children of the future. This book is as much a gift to the mokopuna (grandchildren) of Maata Wharehoka as it is for the world. It is our task, as adults, to build a world informed by the vision of Te Whiti o Rongomai, Tohu Kākahi, and their followers, Te Ru and Maata Wharehoka.

At the same time, this book aims to transmit a lineage of exceptional women little known to the larger world. Their names are in this text: Te Puea, Eva Rickard, Patricia Grace, Tariana Turia, Rose Pere, Aunty Marj Rau, Sally Karena, Ina Okeroa, and many others, including those whose names I do not know. My apologies to the many I have not mentioned, including the multitude of stalwart kuia in every Māori household. The roots of kuia reverberate back through time into timelessness, and beyond time and space. These indefatigable women are firmly grounded, practical, and in service to their people. These women can stand for Parliament, or build marae, create organizational cohesion, advocate for health, raise children to be proud of their Māori heritage, and take care of babies. This is kuiatanga, the way of the kuia (women elders). Perhaps it should be the title of this book.

This book is also about land. The sense of belonging that Māori have to their whenua, their rivers, mountains, plants, and communities is, it seems to me, what so many people in the world long for and yet cannot quite comprehend. The rapacious land theft by the British, which has such thunderous reverberations throughout history, is gut-wrenching, wordlessly and horrifyingly brutal, and irreparable in its magnitude. That Māori, inspired by the modeling of Te Whiti o Rongomai, have carved out a route to peace that is, by my sights, astounding. I am a survivor of sexual assault, domestic violence, and political torture, and it has taken me most of my life to be peaceful and forgiving about this.

What motivated me to want to write this book is my refusal to let Maata's legacy go undocumented. I also want that legacy to go beyond any one location and into the larger world that needs it so desperately. The silence that hangs heavily on the contributions of women, particularly women who prioritize their hard-to-hear truths, must be lifted. I believe this will enlighten the world and open doorways to innovation that remain closed due to patriarchy.

One of the important awakenings for me in writing this book was becoming aware of the lives of precolonial women. I am grateful to Kura Moeahu who, in a conversation I had with him about Maata, pointed me in this direction. Through these investigations, I began to see Maata as a continuation of a long line of empowered, determined, hard-working, and deeply respected women. I saw that Maata embodied the women's leadership that had been completely integrated into precolonial life throughout the world. Recognizing the extent of this lineage, I had to acknowledge the fortifying ancestry sustaining all kuia, crones, and elders, and how this was the source of our resilience.

When asked to speak to their experiences of Maata Wharehoka, many of her peers smile and say, "Some find her hard to take because she is so straightforward. She says what she means, whether you like it or not. She doesn't care what anyone thinks of her. She just voices her truth." The courage of a Māori woman living in a hegemonic world, resurrecting tikanga that has been pushed down by capitalism and land grabs, must be preserved and celebrated. So, too, must her courage in protecting her language and the future of her children, grandchildren, and great-grandchildren from a culture that wants to swallow them up and make them white or invisible be celebrated and maintained. I will not allow it to be secreted away. This is what we need to know to forge a livable future for all our children.

Maata Wharehoka has lived as a resource for Māori girls, women, families, and communities. Te Waka Ruapounamu McLeod, now the Māori Ward Councillor of the New Plymouth District Council, speaks of meeting Maata first as a young girl and "wanting to listen to her, to just sit beside her." Te Waka tells of Maata's role in preparing Wendy Ruapounamu, Te Waka's mother, for Kahu Whakatere when she succumbed to cancer at the age of fifty-one. Te Waka was twenty-two years old then, and Maata, who had been friends with Wendy, who was also a weaver, stepped in and unified the family and the community surrounding them, through Kahu Whakatere, the regenerated tikanga (practice) for death that Maata developed and that is relayed in its own chapter in this book. Tenderly, competently, thoroughly, and lovingly, Maata taught the extended family to weave the whāriki, the mats and robes, for Kahu Whakatere. "It is not only Pākehā who learn from Maata," Te Waka says, "It is also Māori."

Te Waka also speaks of how artfully Maata ensured the circle surrounding Wendy's body was clean, clear, and what Wendy would have wanted. A situation arose where someone from the community did not belong there because of unresolved conflict, but no one had informed Maata about that. Instead, Maata sensed it, with her prescient antennae, and suggested that the group take a thirty-minute break from their weaving and sharing, during which "Anyone who wants to can leave, no questions asked." When the group resumed, that unwelcome person was not among them.

This is the kind of community organizing skill that Maata exudes, giving her an amazing capacity to make things happen in accordance with tikanga. As Te Waka says, "Maata makes everything tikanga," so that in her presence, everyone feels they are participating in a holy ritual. This draws people, over and over, back to Maata and back to Parihaka, where they can soak up the timeless wisdom of the land and the clearcut wisdom of a kuia (female elder). Our longing for kuia wisdom is ineffable, sublimated in a world that suppresses it but pulsates still, waiting to emerge like hot lava from a quiescent volcano.

Bonita Bigham, now on a Fulbright scholarship at the University of Hawaii at Manoa to research, study, and document Indigenous approaches to honoring the bodies of endangered species that die on Native land, such as on the coasts of Aotearoa, remembers meeting Maata. Bonita, like Te Waka, went to Parihaka with her mother when Bonita was a child. She witnessed how Maata and Te Ru helped to restore Parihaka from its desultory and abandoned condition, repopulated it, and realigned it with its original purpose. Bonita recalls the births of Puna, Ngahina, and Te Akau at Parihaka, and she remembers how irresistibly she was drawn to Maata's magnetic presence. When her mother, Hine Waito, witnessed the Kahu Whakatere of Te Ru Wharehoka, she grabbed her daughter's arm and declared with fierce clarity, "I want that." Maata not only officiated at Hine's Kahu Whakatere, she taught the process to her community, and from that exposure, other communities came to learn this reborn tikanga (practice).

Bonita says that her ongoing contact with Maata, who was the celebrant at Bonita's marriage, elevates her. "Maata will challenge you and make you better. That's life with Maata. That's living with Maata, loving with Maata, laughing with Maata." Just as artist Eliot Collins, husband of Te Waka McLeod says, "Maata is a weaver of people," so Bonita reports that Maata will, as if speaking from a vision that is imperceptible to anyone else, link one person with another, or make a joke that suddenly unites an entire gathering in the spirit of their common and joyful purpose.

This is how Maata Wharehoka has naturally, organically built movements, uplifted women, launched organizations, hosted summits, unified disparate groups, created educational and healing circles, and touched and energized thousands upon thousands of people. Maata Wharehoka is a community organizer, a networker, par excellence. She not only knows instinctually how to do this, she just does it with no fanfare. She does not articulate the inner workings of her mind, which are likely impossible to put into language because of how innately they emerge from within her.

This is why those of us who have seen Maata in action are asked to document her achievements for her. She is unlikely to do that. We are the ones who can record the pedagogy of her artistry, the impacts of her prescience, so that others can learn and be encouraged. We must acquire Maata's skills now, when the compassionate and inclusive actions of communities will save lives and forge a future for humanity. This is why Maata's leadership is the orienting principle of this book.

As young Māori girls, Te Waka McLeod and Bonita Bigham were unforgettably touched by Maata's commanding presence. They wanted something of that, and they got it. They absorbed the juice of Maata's elixir that is made from Māori women's precolonial stature in life, and they found their place in the world with that flowing within them. Bonita and Te Waka, like many others, carry Maata's legacy forward in a multitude of forms. Whether advocating for the honoring of the sacred bodies of whales that wash up on the coast of their iwi and Hapūs or fighting for Māori housing and land rights, Māori place names, rights of nature, Te Reo in the schools, and correct Te Reo pronunciation, Māori women who sat next to Maata Wharehoka—who watched her and listened to her, wove with her or sang with her—carry a piece of her light, her determination, her clarity, and it can never be displaced. As I write this, Te Waka is pregnant with her first child, and that child is receiving, cellularly, the transmission that flows in Te Waka's blood from her mother and from Maata. This power is indestructible. This book shares it with you.

IN MEMORIAM

The Undying Legacy of Maata Wharehoka

December 22, 1950—February 2, 2025

Maata Wharehoka died before her time. Her inspired lineage transmission of wisdom, skill, and dedication deserved a broader audience and a more sustained delivery. This book is an attempt to disseminate her essential teaching, embodied in her actions and words, in every work of art she created, every speech and teaching she delivered, and especially in her manifestation of Kahu Whakatere, the ceremonies and harakeke weavings for dying, death, and burial that she regenerated from Māori tikanga (tradition).

Though she was wracked by pain in her final years and walked trailed by the cords of her oxygen tank, we witnessed her relentless will to live on, fed by her stalwart, fierce spirit. I had the privilege of supporting Maata as I could with healing touch, by writing this book, and by documenting her passionate devotion to her tupuna (ancestors), for women's empowerment, for the unity of all people, for peace, for the protection (manaaki) of future generations and the land, for Taranaki Maunga (Mt. Taranaki), and for Parihaka, the iconic marae where she lived, nestled at the feet of Taranaki Maunga.

My love and respect for Maata Wharehoka will never die. Her humor, her straightforward, insistent and commanding way of being, her delights in the natural world, her ukelele playing accompanied by song, her poetry, her inventiveness and artistry, and her love for her children and her mokopuna, her grandchildren, are some of the variegated strands in the colorful tapestry of Maata's life. They come together with grace, elegance, and indestructible strength, like the harakeke that she wove so skillfully with her hard-working hands.

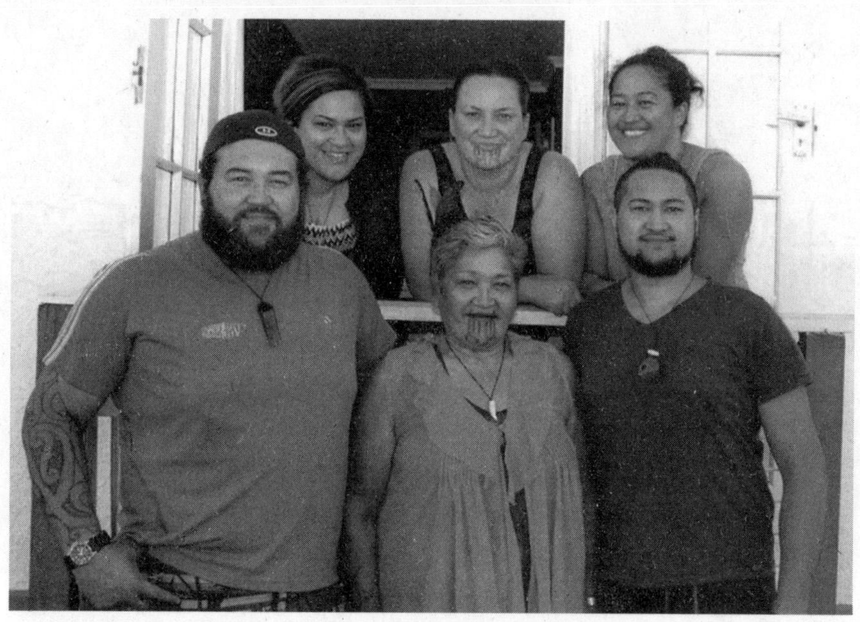

Wharehoka family portrait

AFTERWORD

Unity Is the Way Forward

He maru ahiahi kei muri te maru awatea, he paki arohirohi kei mua.
After the shades of darkness comes the dusk of dawn, whilst before lies the shimmering glory of a fair day.

TE RU KORIRI WHAREHOKA

We are entering a new era when women's voices will be the first we hear, the ones that lead us into the post-colonial world. With the ravages of colonialism and misogyny as teachers that seared our hearts, we can now center feminist and Indigenous wisdom, not deferentially, not by patronizing them, but by recognizing leadership clearly and unequivocally.

Maata Wharehoka was a prophet and a seer. Her unwavering capacity to voice her truth and uphold tikanga Māori never abated. Maata embodied this leadership capacity beginning in her early years, and she never abandoned its promise. Her husband, Te Ru Wharehoka, known tenderly as Papa, saw this. His unique whakataukī (aphorism) epitomizes the new beginning that his wife envisaged, which comes after the dark night of colonialism.

It seems fitting that Maata and Te Ru be recognized not only for their impeccable leadership and representation of tangata whenua but also for the revitalization of Kahu Whakatere. Thanks to them, we can see death not as loss alone but as a portal to true community, which is also what awaits us in the postcolonial world we are building together.

The larger world knows little of Maata and Te Ru Wharehoka. This book intends to correct that. They have been hidden from us, along with countless other Indigenous women and wisdom holders, and it is the joy of this time that we should meet them, hear them, and sit at their feet as they can guide us where we need to go. They, in turn, are always guided by their elders, their tūpuna, their ancestors, who trained them, prepared them, and counseled them devotedly for these times.

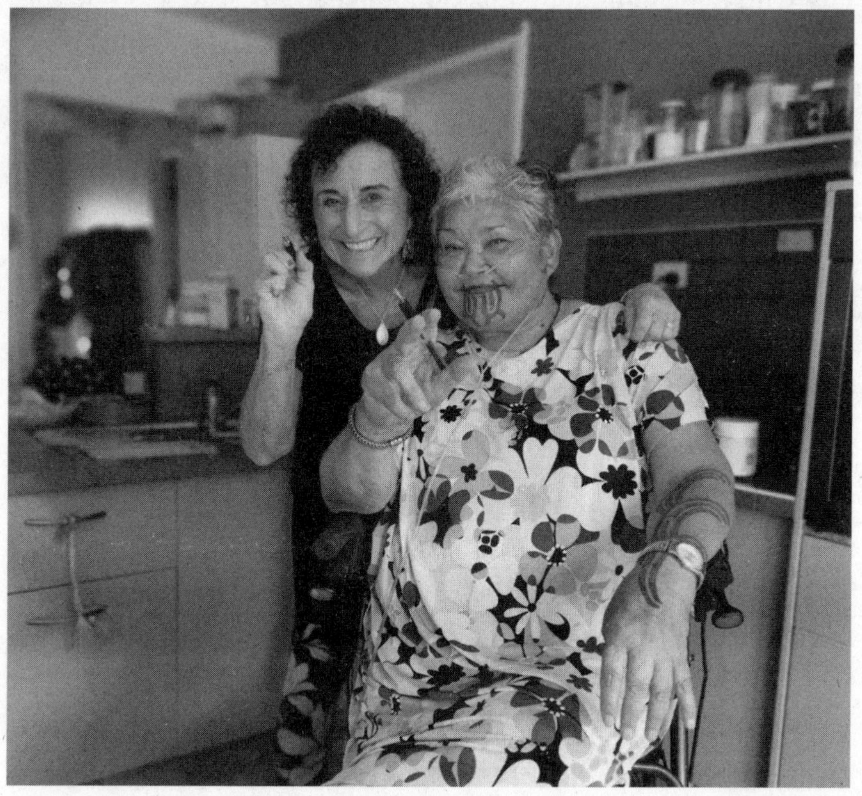

Maata Wharehoka and the author

We are now at an inflection point, a threshold to a transition. We are as if returning from the urupā (burial ground) of hegemony to start a new life in a unified field of dedication to the children of the future.

The intent of this book is to reveal Maata Wharehoka's modeling of empowered womanhood as a message for all people, everywhere. Maata's origins are humble, and though she was revered by everyone who encountered her, she remained unassuming, practical, straightforward, and action oriented. She has shown us that we can be who we truly are and still be a lighthouse to the world.

Why, you may ask, is this book written by a white woman? The answer is that unity is the way forward. Maata chose me, and her family welcomed me to tell Maata's story to the world, because we know that it is only through unity that we can secure a healthy, habitable, and thriving future for our children and grandchildren.

There is great hope in the pages of this book, just as Papa's whakataukī illuminates the shimmering light of a new day. You are that hope. This book, including the questions that follow each chapter, allow us to be the culturally sensitive people we are, so that colonialism and hegemony can be uprooted from our hearts and our minds, and we can step into the original brilliance we were born to embody.

Acknowledgments

It is an honor to have been chosen to write this book. I would like to acknowledge those who believed in me and supported me in doing so. Their encouragement was absolutely sustaining.

Of all of them, the first recognition goes to Rangatira Kuia Maata Wharehoka (Ngāti Tahinga, Ngāti Koala, Ngāti Apakura, Ngāti Toa, Ngāti Kuia). Her faith in me to convey her legacy is humbling.

Jean Hikaka has played a central role by being my ally and liaison, finding treasured documents and photographs, and filling in missing pieces. Time spent with Jean, driving back and forth to Parihaka, being there together, and sharing our insights, has been a treasure of friendship and collaboration.

Ngahina and Te Akau Wharehoka spoke to me from their hearts, and the joyful play and engagement of their children at Parihaka was a special gift to me.

Elias Lilo's presence as well as his commentary were irreplaceable contributions. Puna Aroha shared not only her wisdom and passion about Te Reo, she also shared her students with me. They allowed me to be an audience as they sang songs that Puna had composed, while following her lead in dancing and haka she choreographed.

Hotukura Wharehoka transmitted her love and her wisdom, through her ground-breaking doctoral thesis, and her insights into Māori naming practices and their role in cultural sovereignty.

Kura and Ngapera Moeahu are true educators, mentors, and guides. Speaking with them resonated long after our conversations and wove me into Te Ao Māori in a way that has changed me forever.

Bonita Bigham has been a generous contributor at one of the busiest times of her life when she was transitioning to Hawaii to complete her doctorate.

Te Waka McLeod and Eliot Collins were extremely generous with their time and perceptions.

I also want to thank Ruth Pfister who helped me in a multitude of ways. Her friendship and council are deeply nourishing.

I acknowledge here, with appreciation, the cheery assistance I was the beneficiary of at the Puke Ariki Library in New Plymouth. I practically lived in the Taranaki Research Centre for at least three months, and the staff accommodated me kindly and assisted whenever they could to find books and documents and assured me that I had the reproductions I needed to write this book.

Finally, I would like to thank my husband Robert E. Yuhnke, who supported me completely in this project, even when it involved us being in different parts of the world during important family times, like anniversaries, birthdays, and major holidays. He kept the family together while I did research, and still had the time, despite his own demanding professional life, to share his perspectives and comments about the writing I showed him. He felt the importance of this legacy and knew firsthand the significance of Maata's life and of Parihaka.

Most importantly, I bow in gratitude to the tūpuna who guide me toward sharing the wisdom of Maata Wharehoka and her lineage with the world at a time when it is medicine for all peoples.

Glossary

Aotearoa: New Zealand

Atua: Ancestor with continuing influence; deity.

awhi rito: Parent leaves on the harakeke plant.

haka: Ceremonial or choreographed dance; prelude to battle.

hapū: Regional group.

harakeke: New Zealand flax. A native plant with long, stiff, upright leaves and red flowers. There are many varieties of this plant.

hūmārie: Humility.

ingoa: Name.

iwi: Tribe.

kahu: amniotic sac.

kai: To eat, food, a meal.

kaitiaki: Leadership; caretaker/guardian.

kaitiakitanga: The action or behavior of a leader.

karakia: Incantation, chant, prayer.

karanga: Ceremonial welcome call, usually to welcome visitors onto a marae.

kōhanga: Nest.

kōkohurangi: Tree daisies.

kōrero: Storytelling; dialogues.

kuia: Grandmother, female elder.

kuikui: Matriarchal or kuia-like, elder-like.

kūmara: Sweet potato.

kupu: Word, message.

mahi: Efforts, work.

mana: Spiritual power. Authority through spiritual power. Stewardship. Indestructible power to protect resources.

manaaki: To support, protect, show respect and care for others.

manaakitanga: Gracious generosity.

Māori: Indigenous people of Aotearoa.

marae: The open area in front of a settlement or complex where people live and meet. The word can also be used in reference to the entire complex, such as the Parihaka marae.

maunga: Mountain or mountain peak, such as Mount Taranaki.

mauri: Life force. Vital essence.

moko kauwae: Female lip and chin tattoo.

moko papa: A ceremony for receiving the moko kauwae (chin tattoo for women) and mataora (facial tattoo for men).

mokopuna: Grandchild or grandchildren.

muka: Flax fibers.

Pākehā: Europeans.

papakāinga: Original home. Communal land.

Papatūānuku: Earth. Earth Mother. Wife of Rangi-nui. All living things originate from them.

Parihaka: Epic landmark site in Taranaki, on the North Island of Aotearoa, where in 1881, led by Te Whiti o Rongomai and Tohu Kākahi, the first nonviolent protest was enacted in the face of brutal colonization. Home of Maata Wharehoka.

Parihakatanga: Parihaka consciousness.

poi: A light ball on a string of varying length which is swung or twirled rhythmically to song accompaniment. The verb use of this word is to swing or toss up and down.

pōwhiri: Welcoming ceremony.

pūkenga: Skill.

rangatira: Highly ranked person.

Ranginui: Sky Father.

rongoā: Māori medicine.

tamariki: Youth or children.

tamariki whāngai: Adopted or foster children.

tā moko: The art of Māori tattooing.

tangata whenua: People of the land.

tangi: Mourning, weeping, rite for the dead, funeral. Short for: tangihanga.

tangihanga: Burial. One of the most important rituals of Māori society, usually held on marae. Greenery is the traditional symbol of death.

Te Ao Hurihuri: The ever-turning world.

Te Ao Māori: Māori worldview.

Te Ao Mārama: World of understanding.

Te Ika a Māui: The North Island of Aotearoa/New Zealand.

Te Reo: Language.

teiria: Dahlias.

tiakitanga: Stewardship.

tikanga: Protocol or procedure. Correct way of doing something.

tīpuna: Variation of tūpuna, ancestor, grandparent.

tohunga: Expert, skilled, trained person.

tūpuna: Ancestors.

tūpuna tāne: Grandfathers, male ancestors.

tūpuna wahine: Female ancestors.

urupā: Cemetery.

wahine: Woman, female, feminine.

waiata: Song or to sing; lament.

wānanga: Educational center.

whakaora: Restore to health; revive. To save. To heal. Can also be healing or restoring.

whakaruruhau: A haven.

whakatere: To navigate.

whānau: Family. Kinship.

whare: House, building, residence.

wharenui: Meeting house, main building, or main room.

whare tangata: Womb; the home of the people.

whāriki: To cover with a mat; ground covering or mat.

whenua: Placenta; land.

WHAKATAUKĪ

Proverbs/Aphorisms

The proverbs or aphorisms that are woven into everyday Māori conversation, speechmaking, and cultural and educational settings are a unique literary phenomenon, totally dissimilar to their Westernized counterparts.

They are like medicinal modules, aligning the listener with destiny and heritage. They arise from the timelessness that is innate in Te Ao Māori, the Māori worldview. Each aphorism is like a fiber from a harakeke plant, unifying and organizing in collective and individual spheres. Whakataukī are self-fulfilling. Even in my attempt to define whakataukī here, I am relying on them to guide me.

Whakataukī are motivational, inspirational, problem-solving droplets. They are poetic, pithy, and unifying. They are antidepressants, delivered in microdoses whenever needed. Their origins are usually unknown, but I feel safe to suggest that whakataukī are voices of tūpuna.

Whakataukī reconnect us to purpose. They are solution-based, life-affirming recipes. Like koans or haiku, they require that we stop, pause, reflect, come to center, and act from their wisdom transmission.

The whakataukī collected here are a very small sampling of the vast wisdom stream that exists and that continues to rain down like mana to uplift us all.

He aha te mea nui o te ao? He tangata. He tangata. He tangata.
What is the most important thing in the world? It is people. It is people. It is people.

He tūpuna, he mokopuna.
We are all ancestors; we are all grandchildren.

Kia whakatōmuri te haere whakamua.
I walk backward into the future with my eyes fixed on the past.

He ora te whakapiri, he mate te whaka ta riri.
There is strength in unity, defeat in anger.

Manaaki whenua, manaaki tangata, Haere whakamua.
Care for the land, care for the people, go forward.

He kai kei aku ringa.
There is food at the end of my hands.

Ka pu te ruha ka hao te rangtahi.
As an old net withers, another is remade.

Kia kaha, kia māia, kia Manawatu.
Be strong, be brave, be steadfast.

Whāia te iti Kahurangi, ki te tuohu koe, me he maunga teitei.
Seek the treasure that you value most dearly; if you bow your head, let it be to a lofty mountain.

Whiria te tangata.
Weave the people together.

Na koutou I tangi, na tatau katoa.
When you cry, your tears are shed by us all.

Kāore te kūmara a kōrero mo tōna reka.
The kūmara does not speak of its sweetness.

Ahakoa he iti, he pounamu.
Be it ever so small, it is as precious as jade.

He kākano I ruia mai I Rangiātea.
The seed will not be lost.

He wahine he taonga.
Every woman is a treasure.

Ehara taku toa I te toa takitahi, engari he toa takitini.
Our strength is not made from us alone, but it is made from many.

Piki kau ake te whakaropai, haukake tonu iho.
When a good thought springs up, it is harvested. A good idea should be used immediately.

Patua I te taniwha, o te whakamā.
Don't let shyness (or any monster) overcome you.

Kaua e mate wheke mate uroroa.
Strive for your goals by being strong and resilient like a hammerhead shark.

Kua hinga he tōtara i te wao nui a Tane.
A great one has fallen in the forest of Tāne. (Said when a leader has transitioned from this plane.)

Bibliography

Aotea Utanganui (Museum). 2020. *Tales & Tonga of South Taranaki*. Pātea, NZ: Aotea Utanganui Museum of South Taranaki.

Best, Elsdon. 1929. *The Whare Kohanga (the "Nest House") and Its Lore: Comprising Data Pertaining to Procreation, Baptism, and Infant Betrothal, Etc.: Contributed by Members of the Ngati-Kahungunu Tribe of the North Island of New Zealand*. Wellington, NZ: A. R. Shearer.

Bonney, Judith, and Gillian Chapman. 2011. *Ngā Mōrehu: The Survivors: The Life Histories of Eight Māori Women*. Wellington, NZ: Bridget Williams Books.

Brooks, Barbara. 2016. *A History of New Zealand Women*. Wellington, NZ: Bridget Williams Books.

Brown, Amy, ed. 1994. *Mana Wahine: Women Who Show the Way*. Auckland, NZ: Reed Books.

Burton, Graham J., and Abigail L. Fowden. 2015. "The Placenta: a Multifaceted, Transient Organ." *Philosophical Transactions of the Royal Society of London. Series B, Biological Sciences* 370 (1663).

Clarke, Alison. 2012. *Born to A Changing World: Childbirth in Nineteenth-Century New Zealand*. Wellington, NZ: Bridget Williams Books.

Clark, Helen. 2018. *Women Equality Power: Selected Speeches from a Life of Leadership*. Auckland, NZ: Allen & Unwin.

Craig, Dick. 1995. *The Realms of King Tāwhiao: with Review of Causes of 1860–64 Māori Wars*. Tauranga, NZ: D. Craig.

Diamond, Paul. 2003. *A Fire in Your Belly: Māori Leaders Speak*. Wellington, NZ: Huia.

Diamond, Paul. 2007. *Makereti: Taking Māori to the World*. Auckland, NZ: Random House New Zealand.

Duff, Michelle. 2023. *Jacinda Ardern*. Auckland, NZ: Allen & Unwin.

Ellis, Lee, Eshah A. Wahab, and Malini Ratnasingan. 2012. "Religiosity and Fear of Death: A Three-Nation Comparison." *Mental Health, Religion & Culture* 16 (2): 179–99.

Foley, Alfred D. 2004. *Jane's Story: Biography of Heeni Te Kirikaramu/Pore (Jane Foley): Woman of Profound Purpose*. Auckland, NZ: A. D. Foley.

Grace, Patricia. 2021. *From the Centre: A Writer's Life*. Auckland, NZ: Penguin Random House New Zealand.

Grace, Patricia, and Waiariki Grace. 2004. *Earth, Sea, Sky: Images and Māori Proverbs from the Natural World of Aotearoa New Zealand*. Wellington, NZ: Huia.

Grace, Patricia, and Robyn Kahukiwa. 1984. *Wahine Toa: Women of Māori Myth*. Auckland, NZ: Collins.

Greensill, Angeline, Annette Sykes, and Leonie Pihama, eds. 1998. *Tuaiwa Hautai Gerard Rickard, 1925–1997: The Pools*. Whaingaroa, Aotearoa: The Independent State of Transportation: Nine-Born Editation & Moko Productions.

Heuer, Berys. 1972. *Maori Women*. Wellington, NZ: Published for the Polynesian Society by A.H. & A.W. Reed.

Hohaia, Te Miringa, Gregory O'Brien, and Lara Strongman, eds. 2006. *Parihaka: The Art of Passive Resistance*. Wellington, NZ: Victoria University Press.

Hond, Ruakere. 2021. "Parihaka: Remembering November 5, 1881." National Library of New Zealand. Filmed November 5. YouTube, 1:14:50.

Horsfield, Anne K., and Miriama Evans. 1988. *Maori Women in the Economy: A Preliminary Review of the Economic Position of Maori Women in New Zealand*. Wellington, NZ: Ministry of Women's Affairs.

Ihimaera, Witi. 2011. *The Parihaka Woman*. Auckland, NZ: Random House.

Keenan, Danny. 2015. *Te Whiti O Rongomai and the Resistance of Parihaka*. Wellington, NZ: Huia.

King, Michael. 2006. *Te Puea: A Life*. Auckland, NZ: Reed Books.

King, Michael. 1983. *Whina: A Biography of Whina Cooper*. Auckland, NZ: Hodder and Stoughton.

Machado de Oliviera, Vanessa. 2021. *Hospicing Modernity: Facing Humanity's Wrongs and the Implications for Social Activism*. Berkeley, CA: North Atlantic Books.

Maiharoa, Te Keli. 2022. "Kaupapa Maori as Transformative Indigenous Analysis." In *The Routledge International Handbook of Indigenous Resilience*, edited by Hilary N. Weaver. New York, NY: Routledge.

Marya, Rupa and Raj Patel. 2021. *Inflamed: Deep Medicine and the Anatomy of Injustice*. New York, NY: Farrar, Straus and Giroux.

Matata-Sipu, Qiane. 2021. *Nuku: Stories of 100 Indigenous Women*. Mangere, NZ: Qiane Matata-Sipu of QIANE & Co.

McRae, Jane. 2017. *Māori Oral Tradition: He Kōrero Nō Te Āo Tawhito*. Auckland, NZ: Auckland University Press.

Mead, Hirini Moko. 2003. *Tikanga Māori: Living by Māori Values*. Wellington, NZ: Huia.

Miller, Harold. 1966. *Race Conflict in New Zealand: 1814–1865*. Auckland, NZ: Blackwood & Janet Paul.

Mitcalfe, Barry. 1974. *The Singing Word: Māori Poetry*. Wellington, NZ: Price Milburn for Victoria University Press.

Moon, Paul. 2016. *Ka Ngaro Te Reo: Māori Language Under Siege in the Nineteenth Century*. Dunedin, NZ: Otago University Press.

Murchie, Erihāpeti (Elizabeth) Rehu. 1984. *Rapuora: Health and Maori Women*. Wellington, NZ: Maori Women's Welfare League.

Murphy, Ngāhuia. 2014. *Waiwhero, The Red Waters: A Celebration of Womanhood*. Translated by Sean Ellison. Ngaruawahia, NZ: He Puna Manawa Ltd.

Neufled, Hannah Tait, and Jaime Cidro. 2017. *Indigenous Experiences of Pregnancy and Birth*. Bradford, Ontario: Demeter Press.

New Zealand Ministry of Health. 2024. *Tatau Kahakura: Māori Health Chart Book*. 4th ed. Wellington, New Zealand: Ministry of Health.

New Zealand Ministry of Women's Affairs. 1990. *Women and Smoking*. Wellington, NZ: New Zealand Ministry of Women's Affairs.

Nzegwu, Nkiru Uwechia. 2006. *Family Matters: Feminist Concepts in African Philosophy of Culture*. Albany, NY: State University of New York Press.

Paama-Pengelly, Julie. 2010. *Maori Art and Design: A Guide to Classic*

Weaving, Painting, Carving and Architecture. Auckland, NZ: New Holland Publishers.

Paterson, Lachy, and Angela Wanhalla. 2017. *He Reo Wāhine: Māori Women's Voices from the Nineteenth Century*. Auckland, NZ: Auckland University Press.

Pere, Rangimarie Rose. 1997. *Te Wheke: A Celebration of Infinite Wisdom*. Wairoa, NZ: Ao Ako Global Learning New Zealand with the assistance of Awareness Book Company.

Pihama, Leonie. 2018. "Moko Kauae: A Māori Women's Right." *Kaupapa Māori as Transformative Indigenous Analysis* (blog). May 23.

Pihama, Leonie, and Linda Tuhiwai Smith, eds. 2023. *Ora: Healing Ourselves: Indigenous Knowledge, Healing and Wellbeing*. Wellington, NZ: Huia Publishers.

Pihama, Leonie, Marjorie Beverland, Linda Tuhiwai Smith, Ngaropi Raumati, Papahuia Dickson, and Awhina Cameron. 2023. *Taku Kuia E: Honoring Our Grandmothers*. Taranaki, NZ: Tū Tama Wahine o Taranaki Inc.

Puketapu-Hetet, Erenora. 2016. *Maori Weaving with Erenora Puketapu-Hetet*. Wellington, NZ: Hetet Press.

Pullon, Sue, and Cheryl Benn. 2008. *The New Zealand Pregnancy Book: A Guide to Pregnancy, Birth and a Baby's First Three Months*. Wellington, NZ: Bridget Williams Books.

Rameka, Lesley. 2018. "A Māori perspective of being and belonging." *Contemporary Issues in Early Childhood* 19 (4): 367–378.

Rei, Tania, Louise Ormsby, and Anaria Tangohau. 1993. *Maori Women and the Vote*. Wellington, NZ: Huia Publishers.

Rezapour, Mahdi. 2022. "The Interactive Factors Contributing to Fear of Death." *Frontiers in Psychology*, 13 (June).

Sawyer, Jacob S. 2024. "Grief and Bereavement Beliefs and their Associations with Death Anxiety and Complicated Grief in a U.S. College Student Sample." *Death Studies*, 7 (May): 1–12.

Scott, Dick. 2006. *Ask That Mountain: The Story of Parihaka*. London, UK: Raupo/Penguin.

Seed-Pihama, Joeliee Elizabeth. 2017. "Ko wai tō ingoa? The Transformative Potential of Māori Names." Ph.D. diss., University of Waikato.

Sinclair, Shane. 2011. "Impact of Death and Dying on the Personal Lives and Practices of Palliative and Hospice Care Professionals." *CMAJ: Canadian Medical Association Journal* 183(2): 180–87.

Stokes, Evelyn. 2002. *Wiremu Tamihana: Rangatira,* Wellington, NZ: Huia.

Szaszy, Mira. 1993. *Te Tīmatanga Tātau Tātau: Early Stories from Founding Members of the Maori Women's Welfare League.* Edited by Anna Rogers and Miria Simpson (Wahanga Māori). Wellington, NZ: Bridget Williams Books.

Tawhiwhirangi, Iritana. 1992. Interview, June 17. Māori Women's Welfare League.

Te Awekotuku, Ngāhuia. 1991. *Mana Wahine Maori: Selected Writings on Maori Women's Art, Culture, and Politics.* Auckland, NZ: New Women's Press.

Te Awekotuku, Ngāhuia. 2002. "Ta Moko: Culture, Body Modification, and the Psychology of Identity." *The Proceedings of the National Māori Graduates of Psychology Symposium 2002: Making a Difference*, 123–27. Waikato, NZ: University of Waikato.

Te Whāiti, Pania, Mārie B. McCarthy, and Arohia Durie. 1997. *Mai I Rangiātea: Māori Wellbeing and Development.* Auckland, NZ: Auckland University Press.

Wilson, Denise. 2023. "Violence within Whānau and Mahi Tūkino: A Litany of Sound Revisited." PDF file: Te Pūkotahitanga—Tangata Whenua Advisory Group for the Minister of the Prevention of Family Violence and Sexual Violence (March).

Winiata, Whatarangi, 2021. *The Survival of Maori as a People: A Collection of Papers by Emeritus Professor Whatarangi Winiata*, edited by Daphne Luke. Wellington, NZ: Huia.

Index